MW00897769

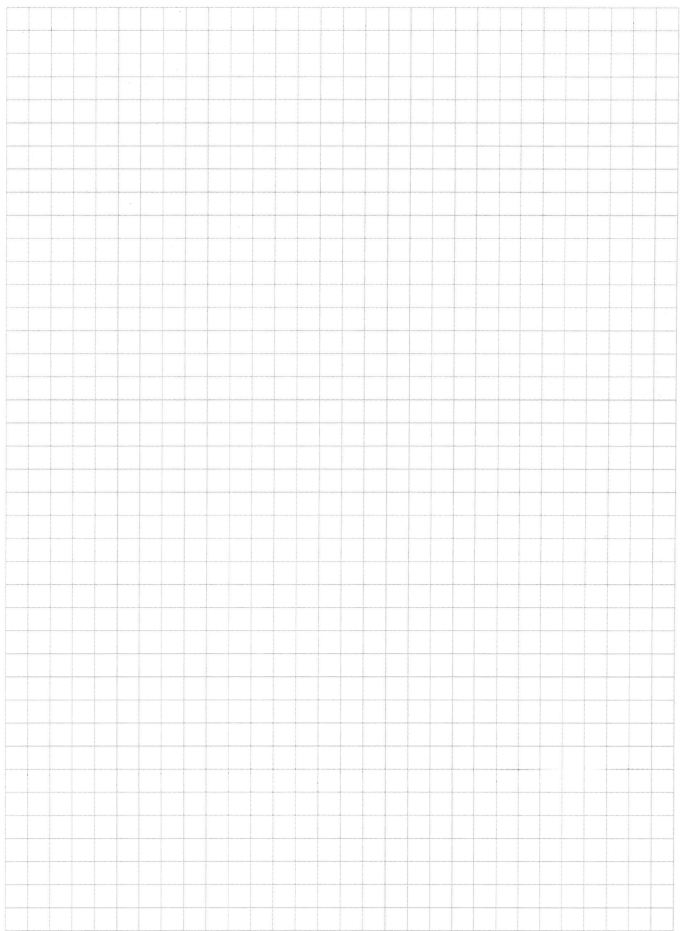

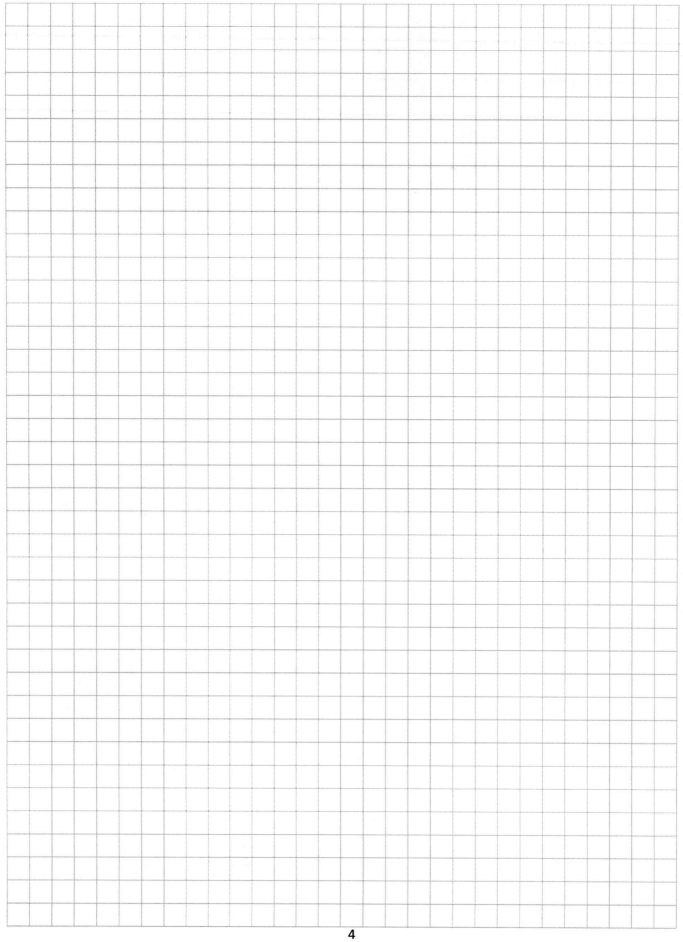

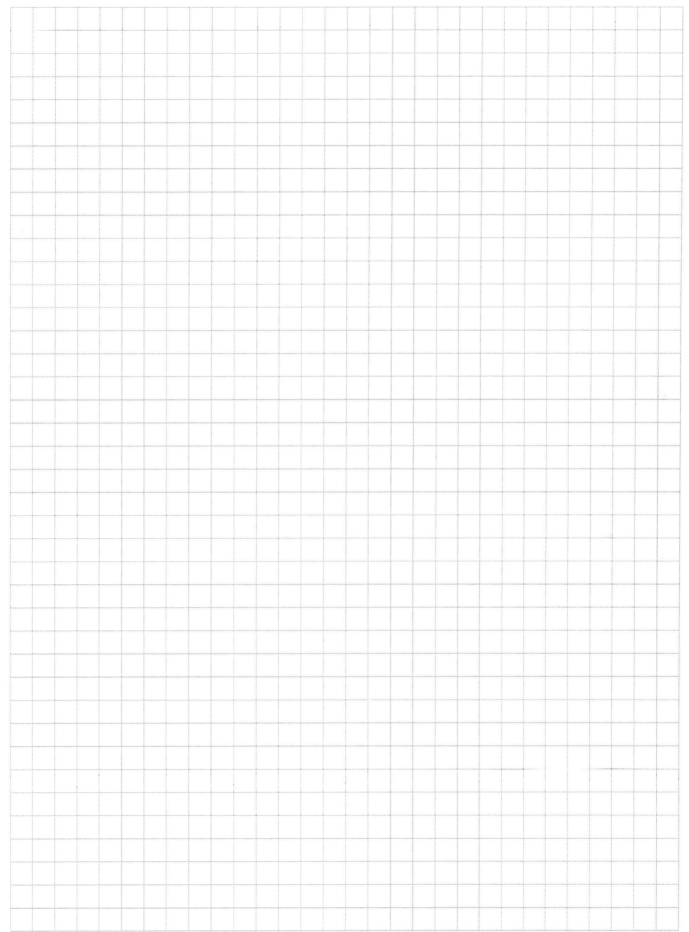

5

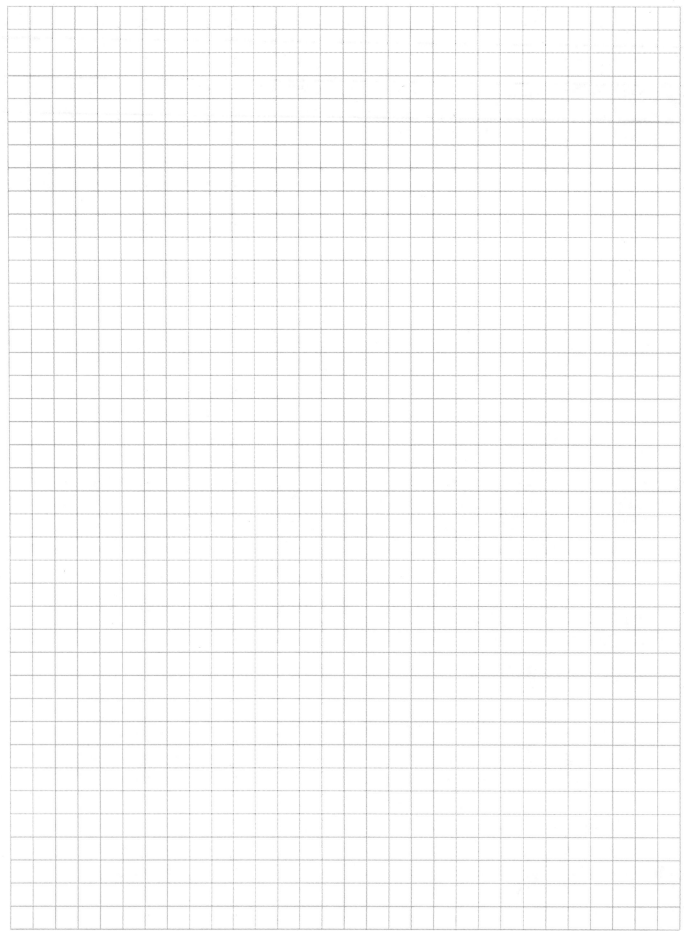

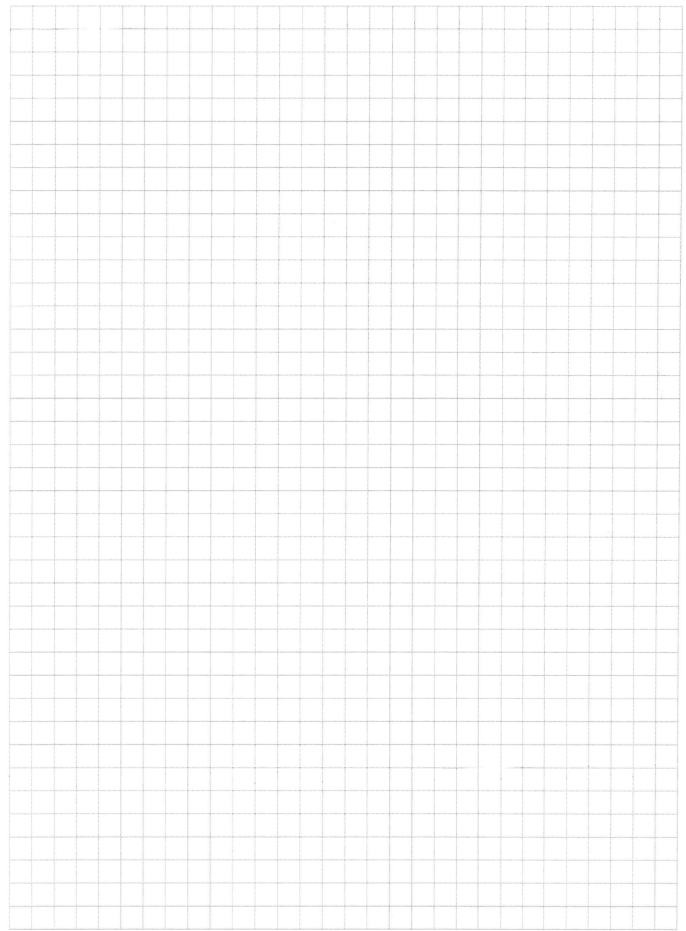

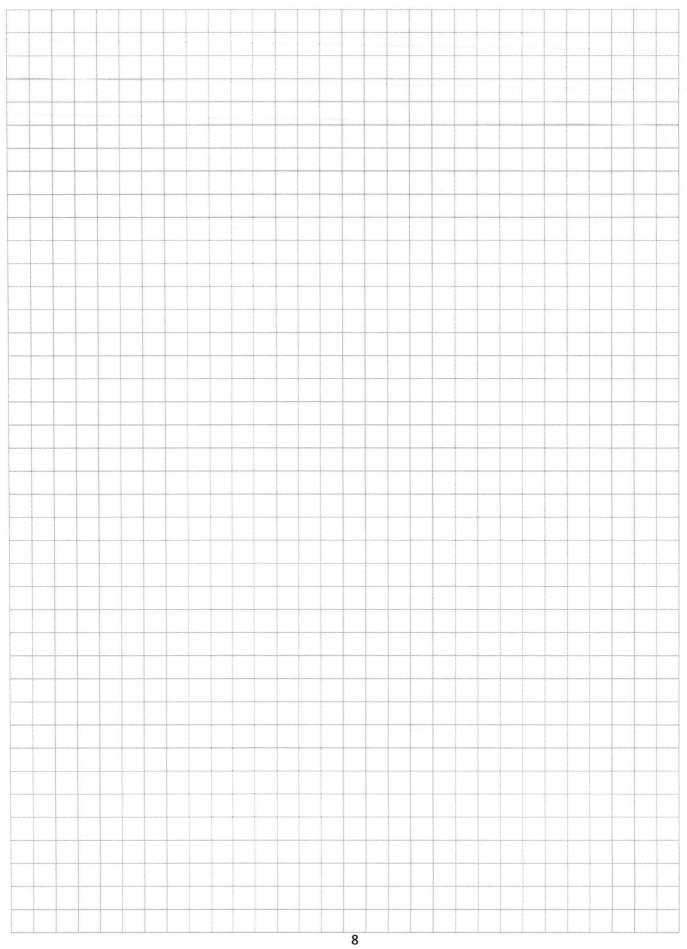

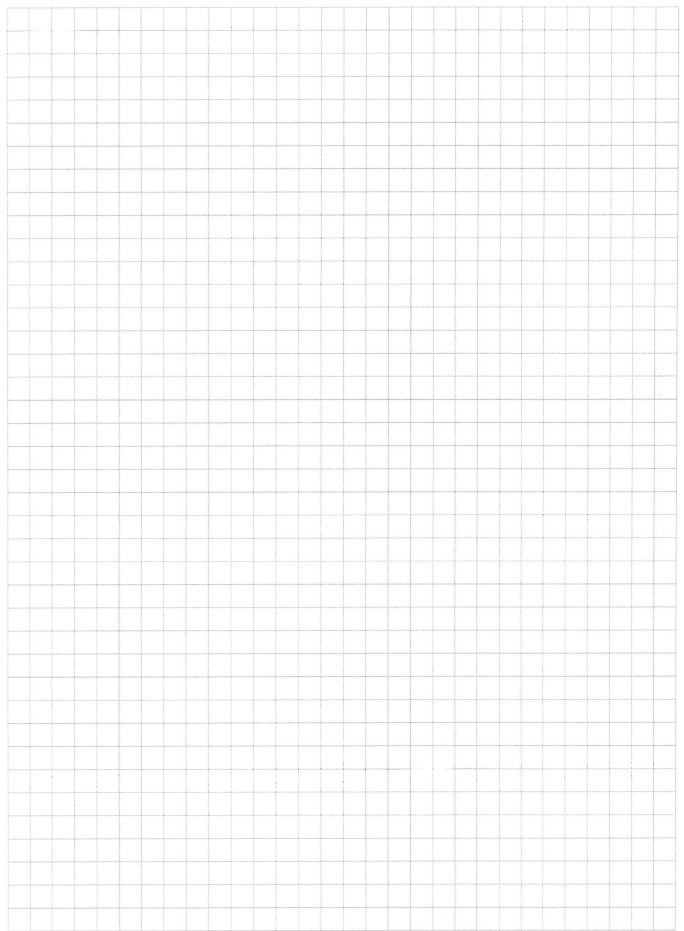

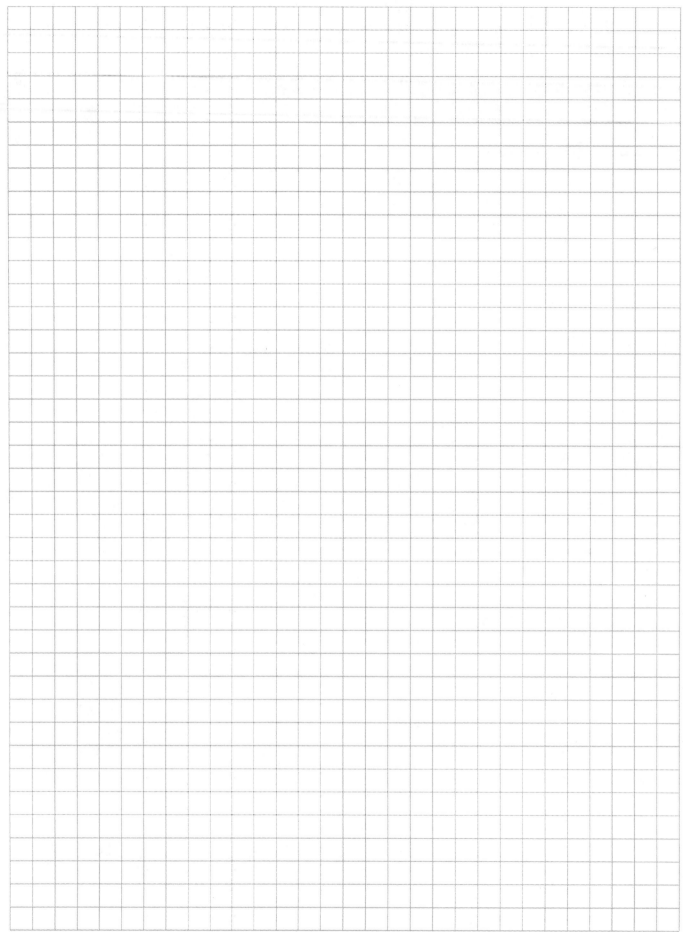

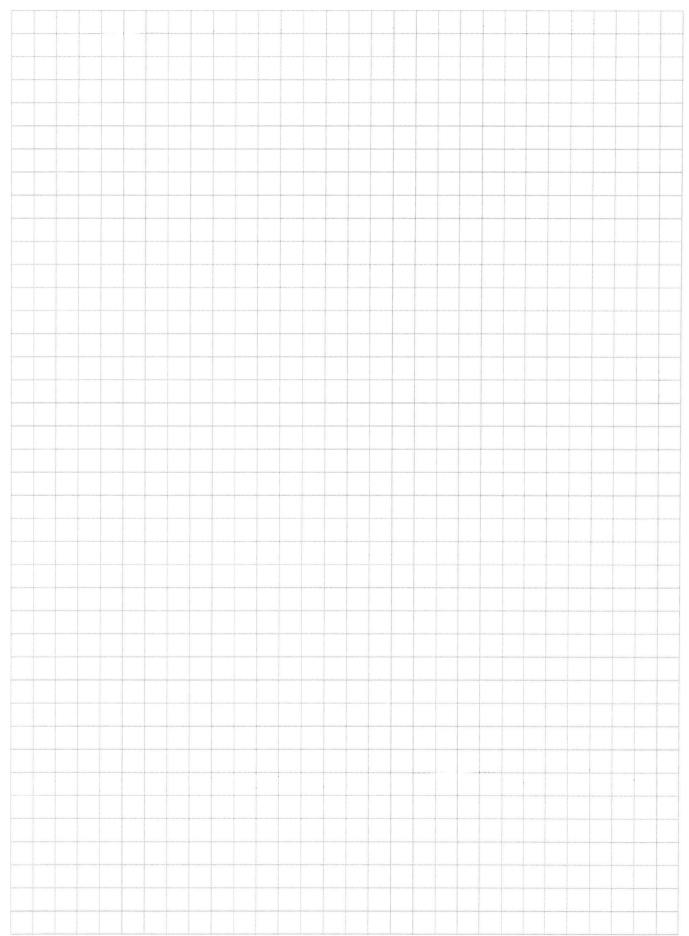

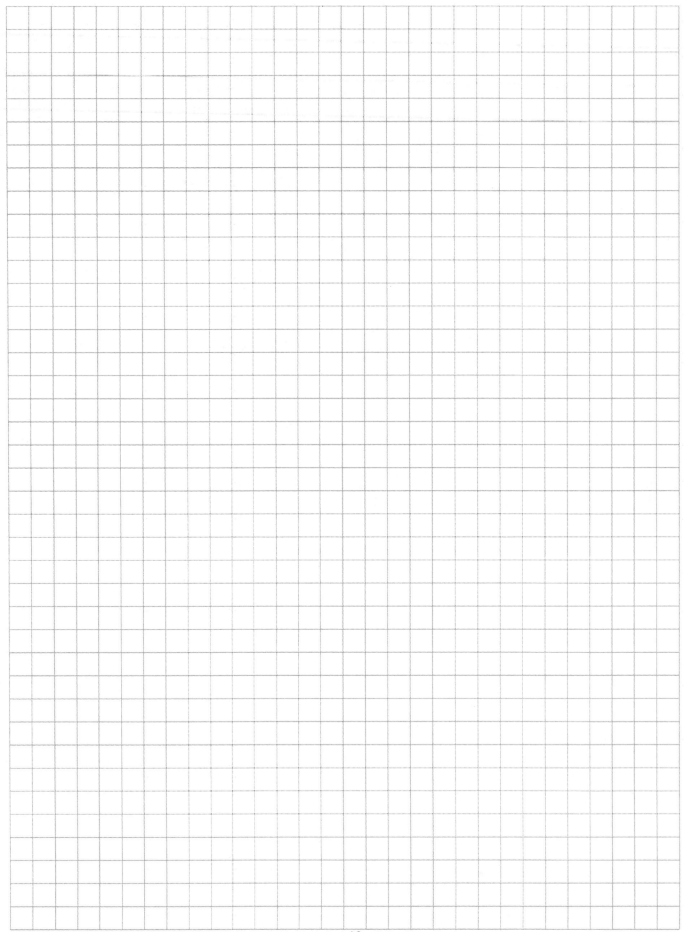

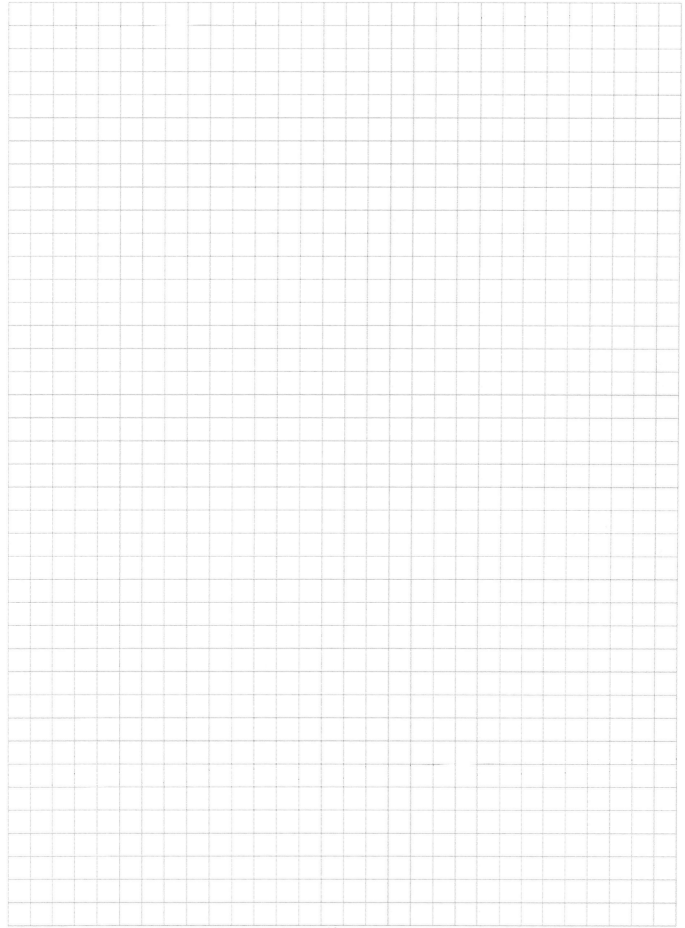

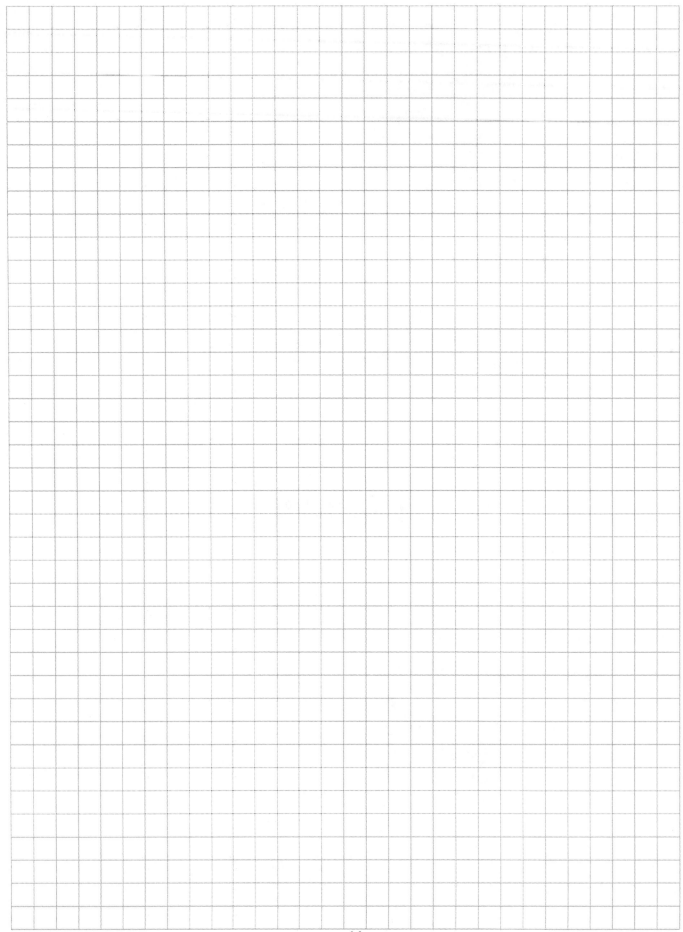

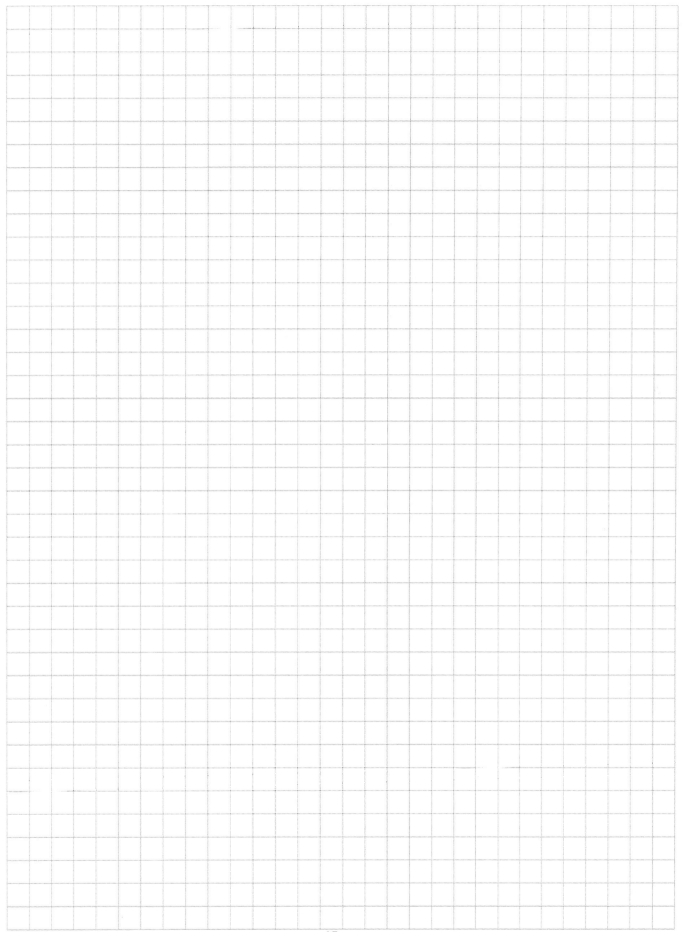

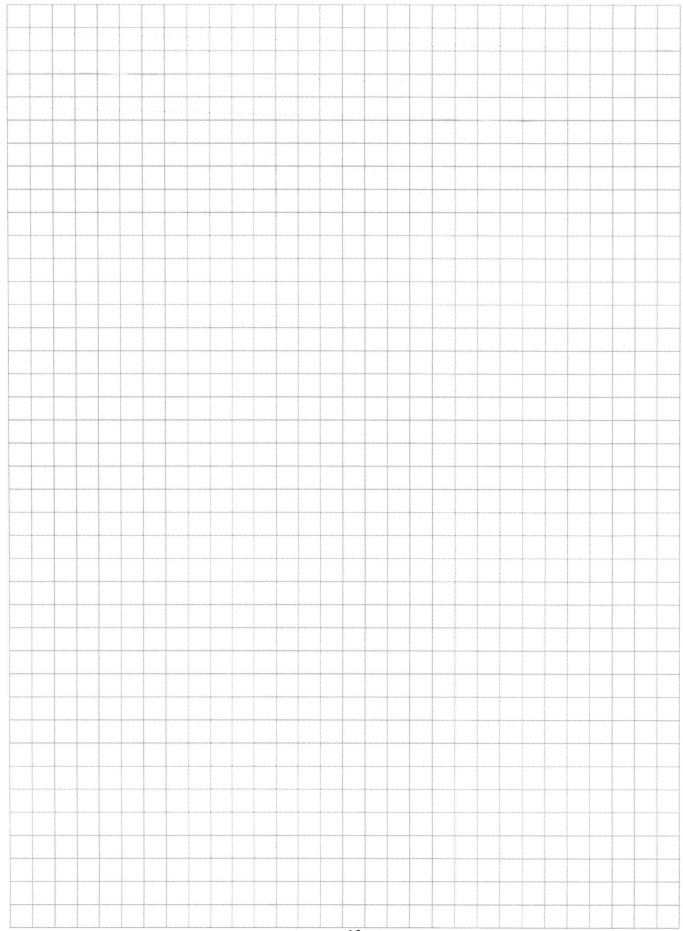

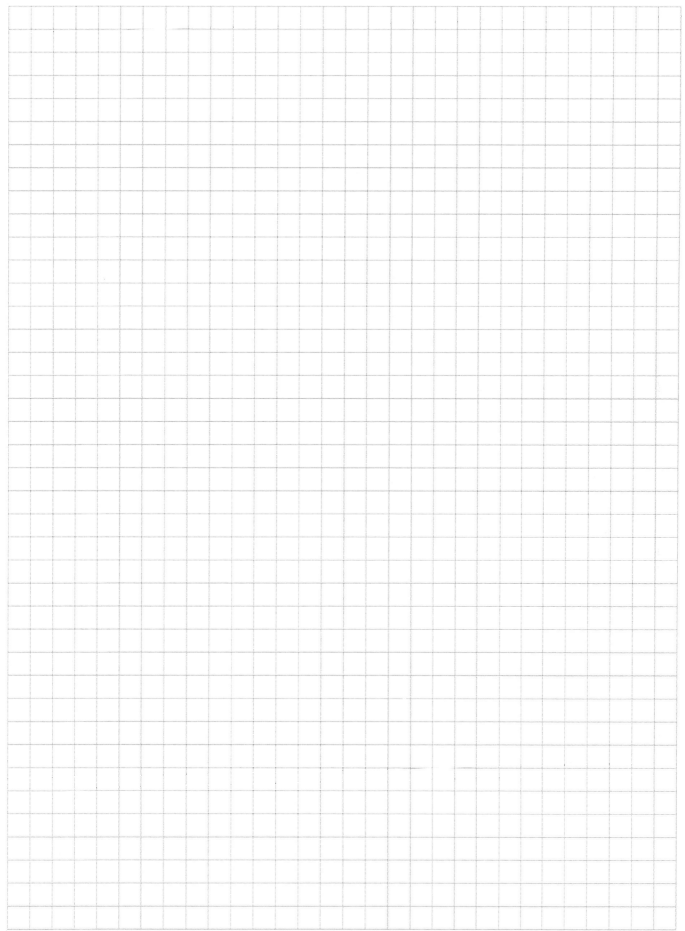

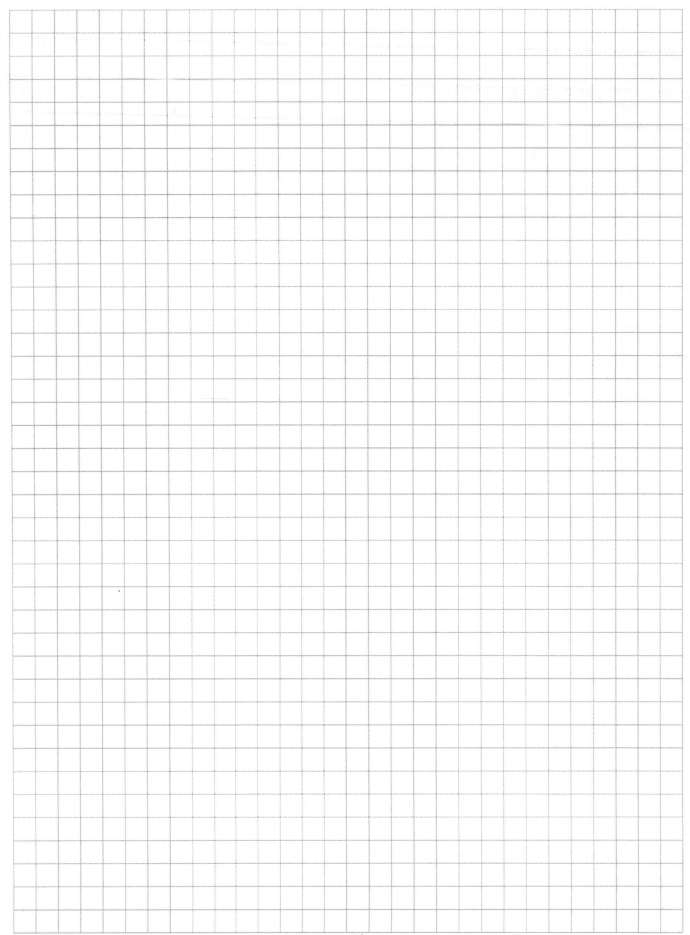

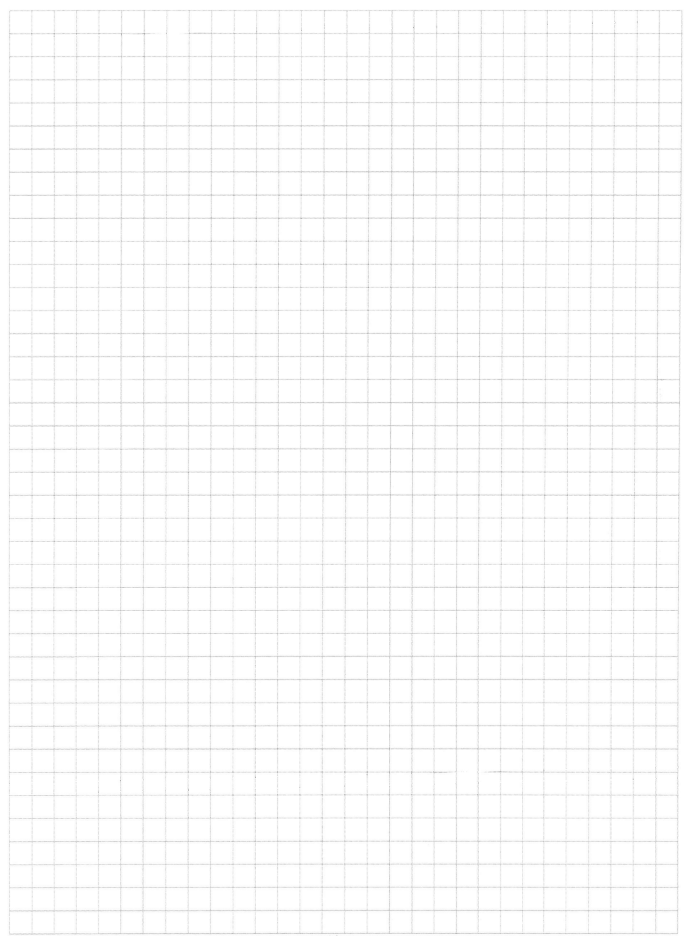

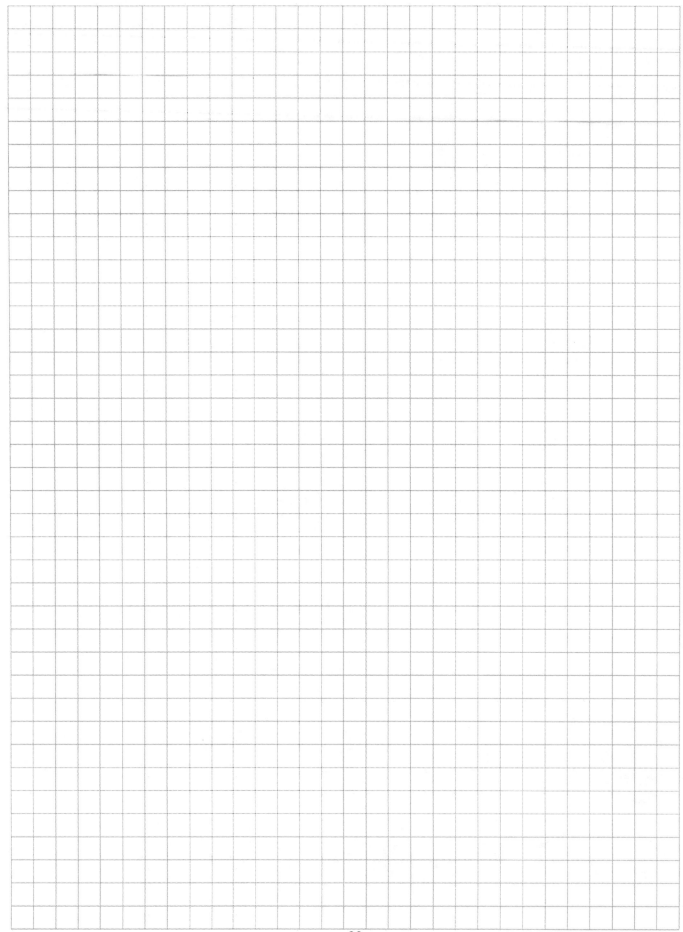

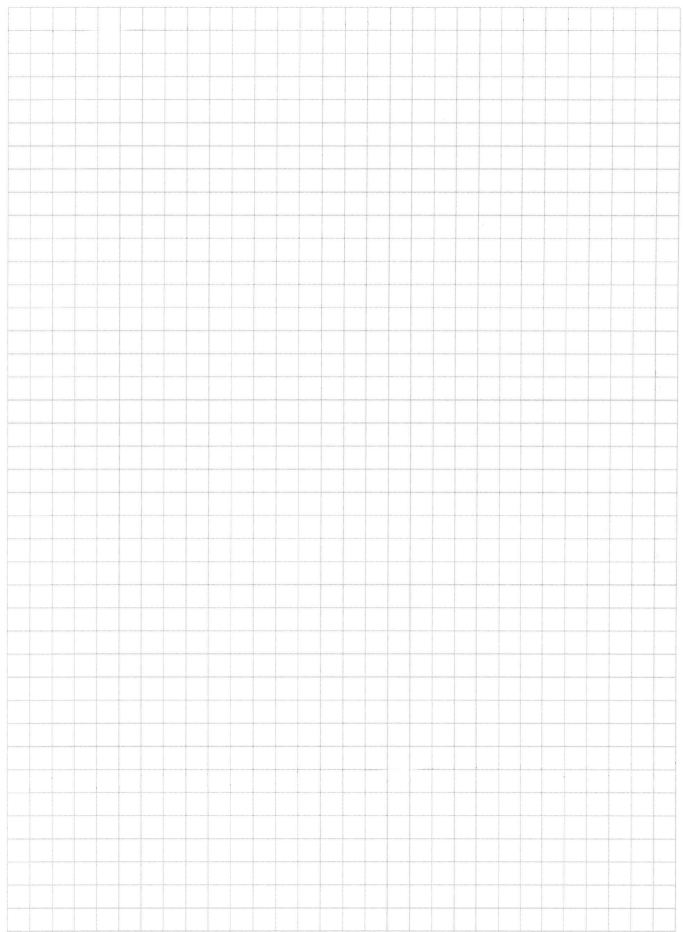

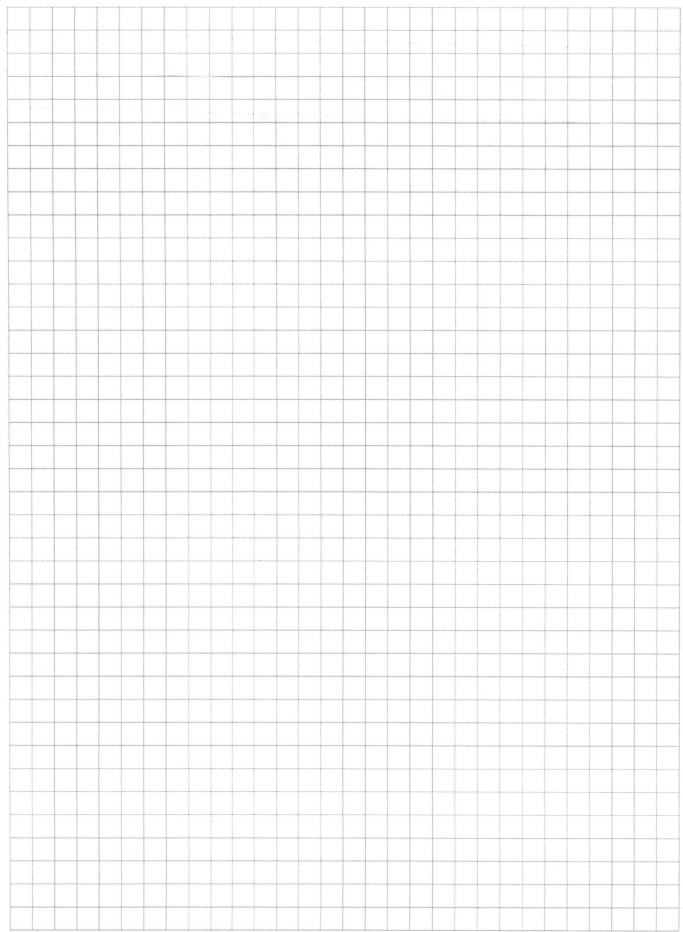

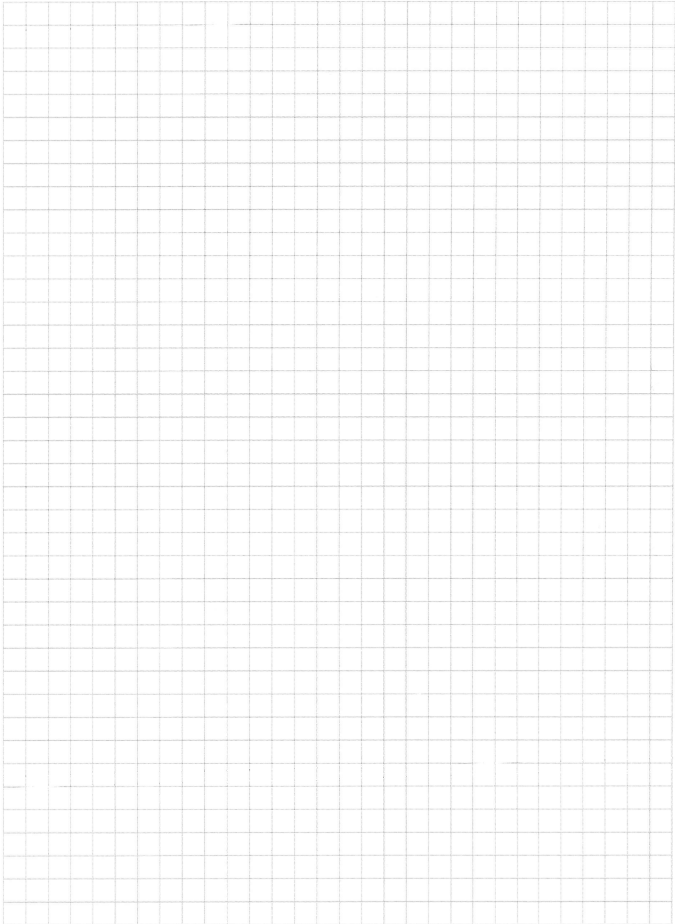

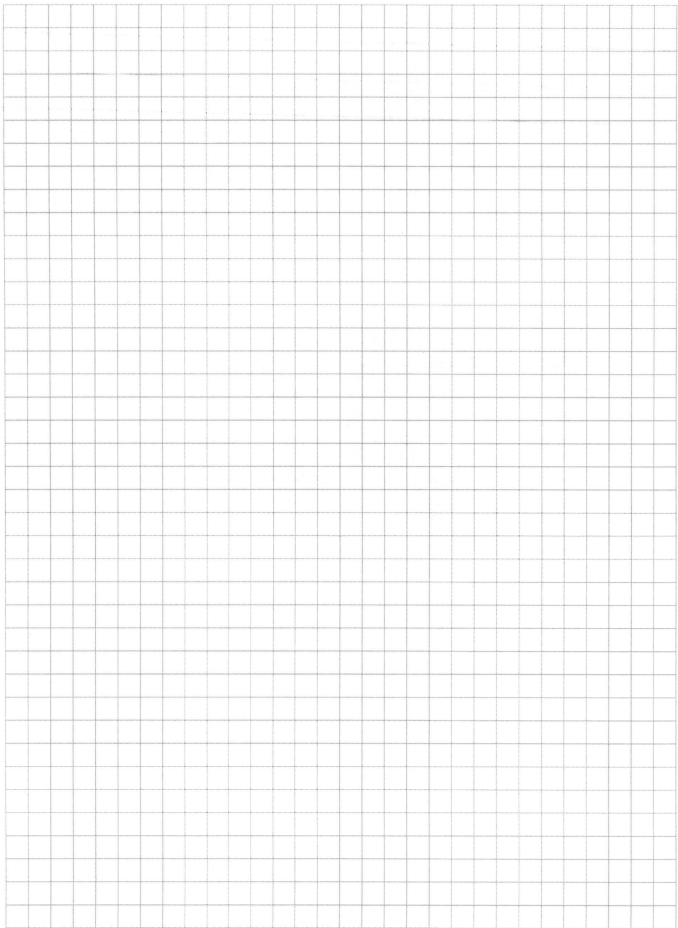

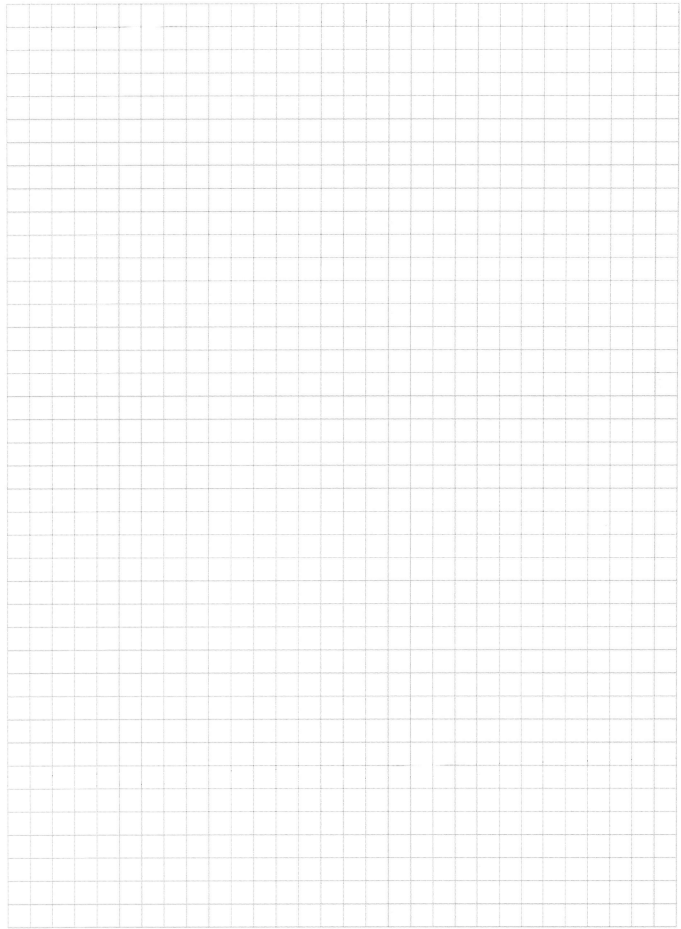

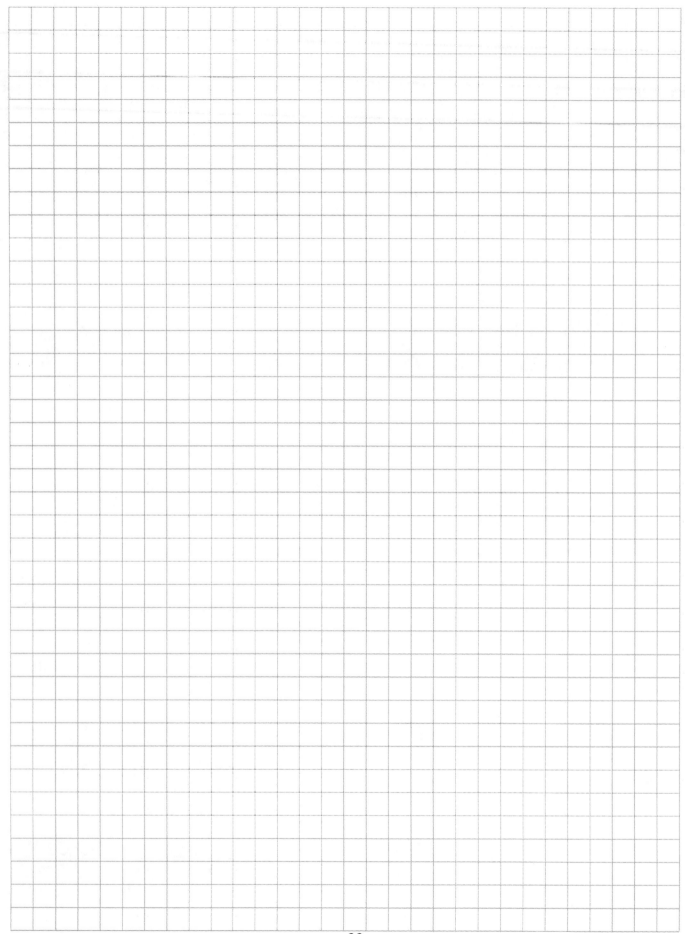

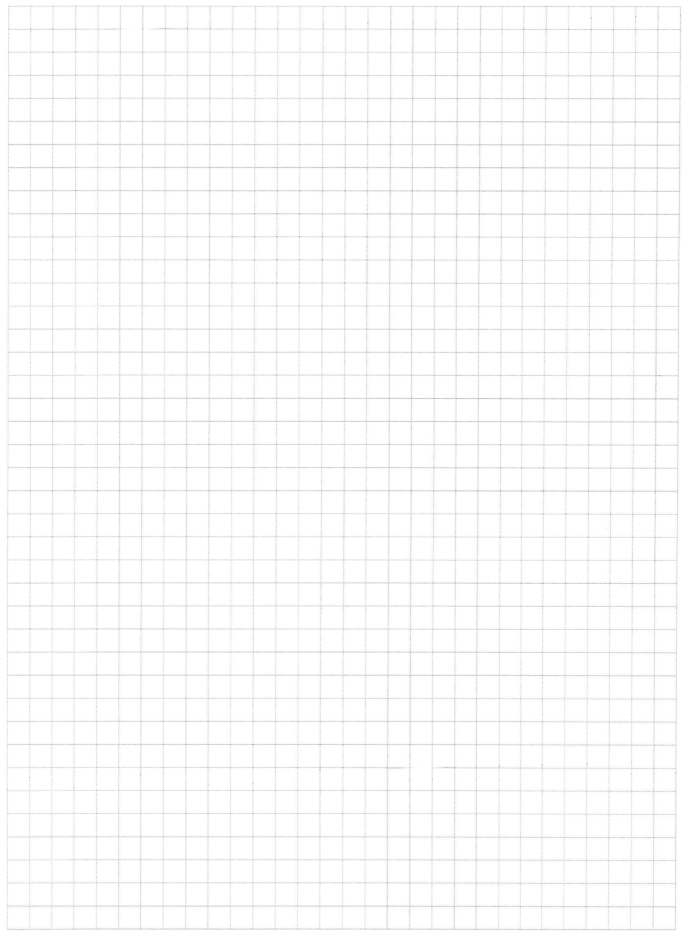

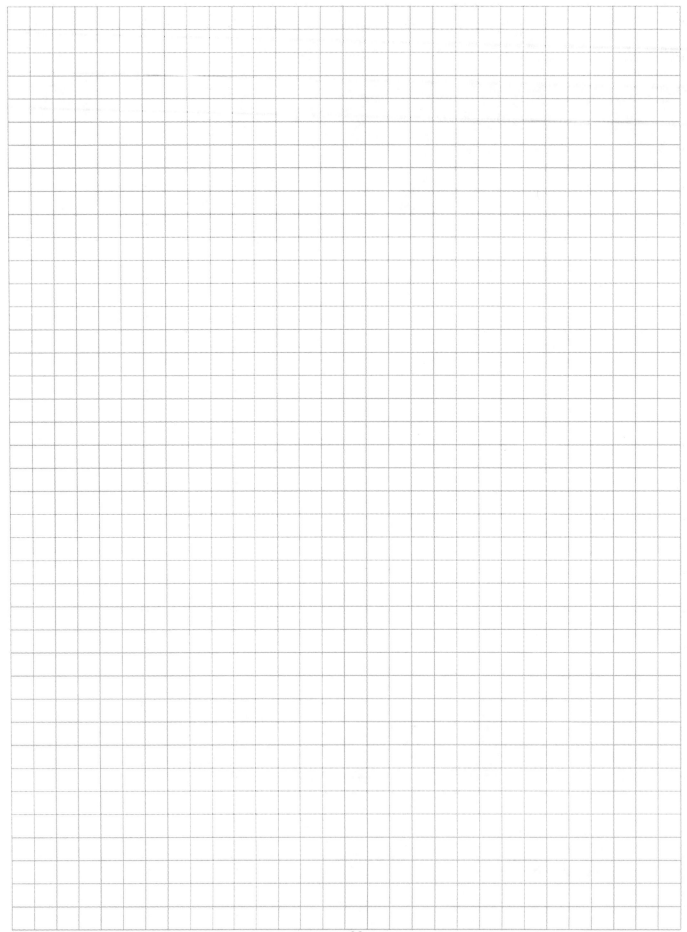

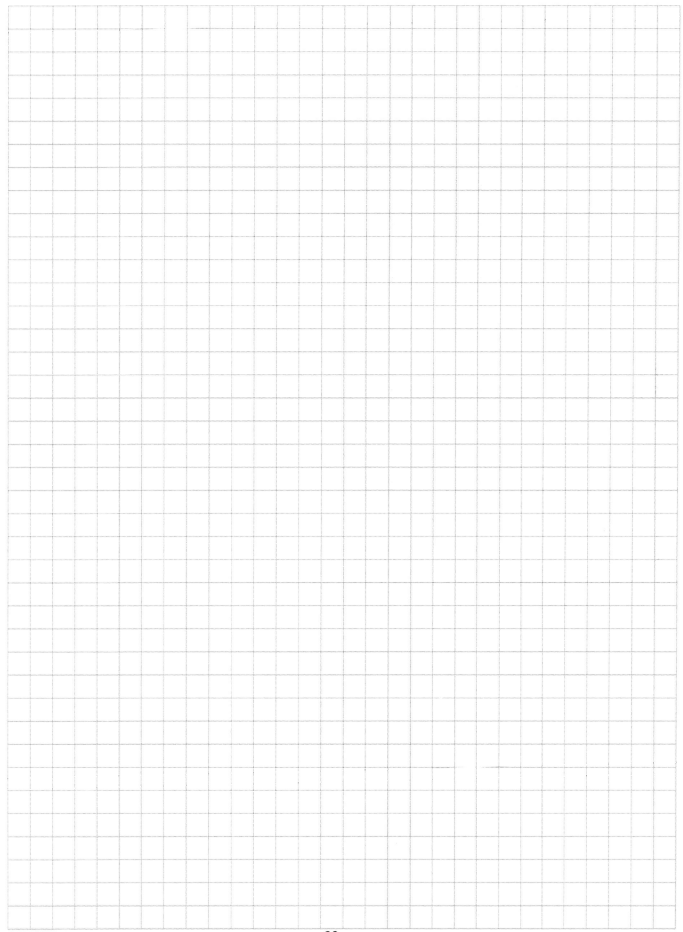

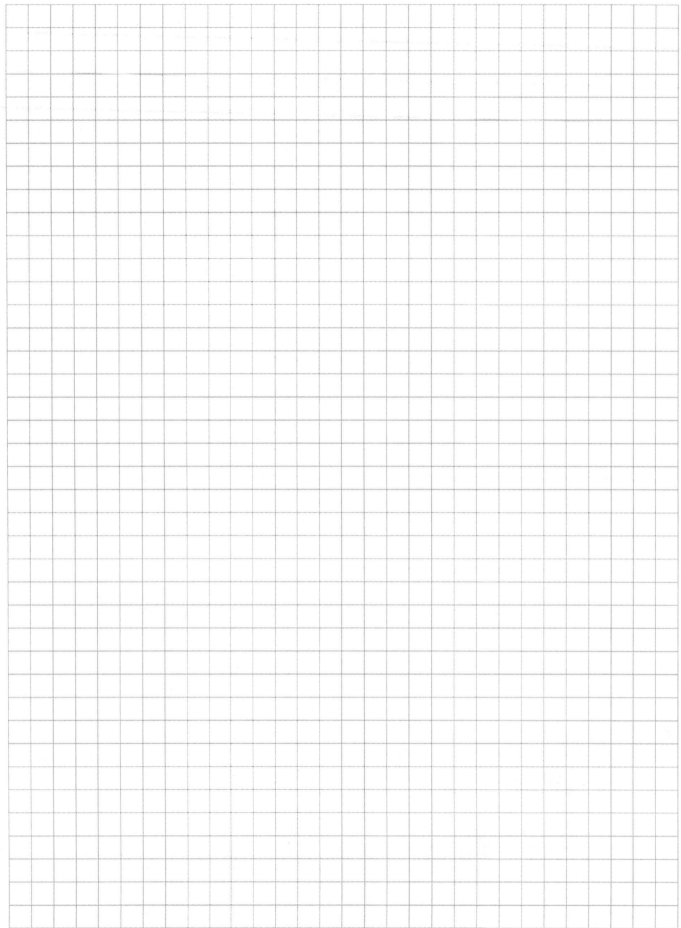

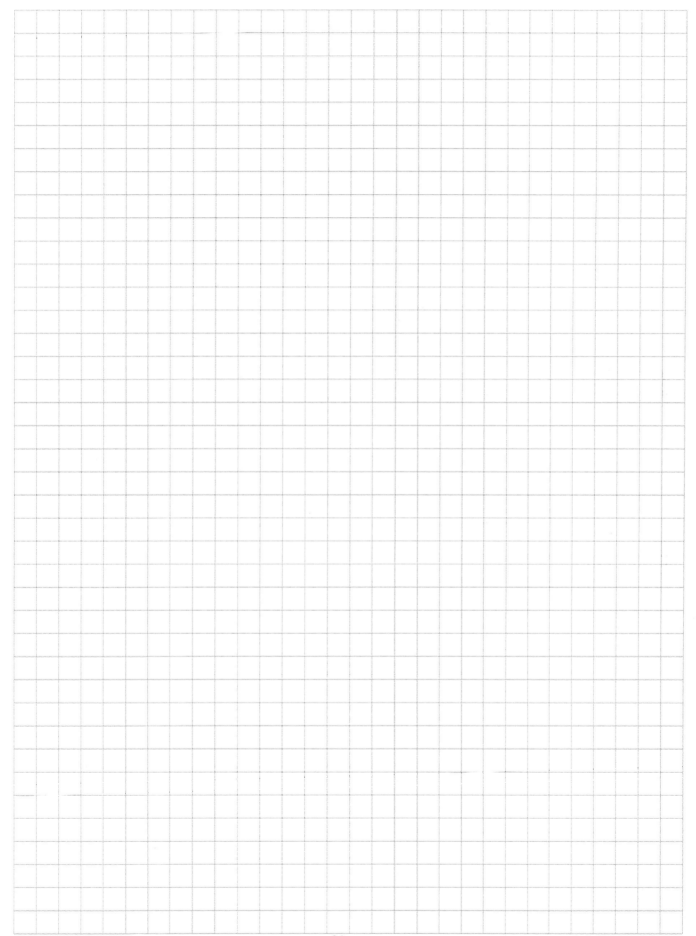

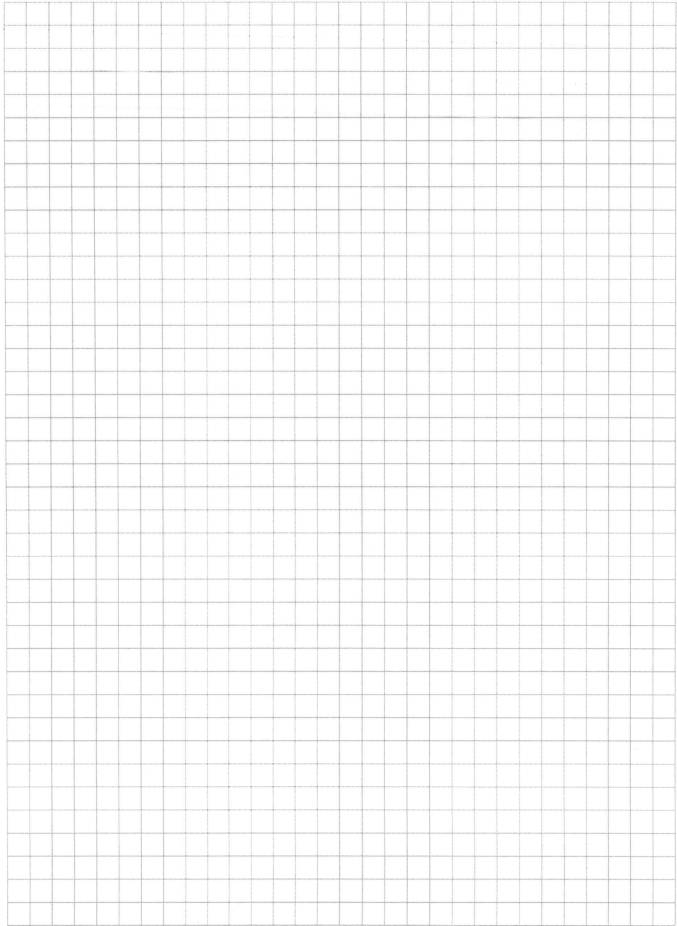

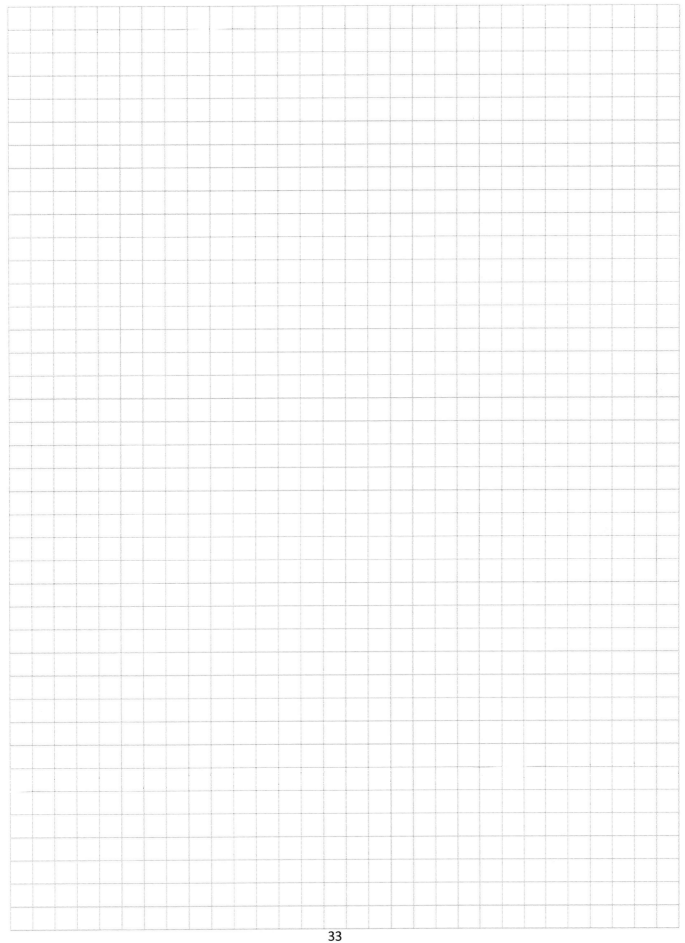

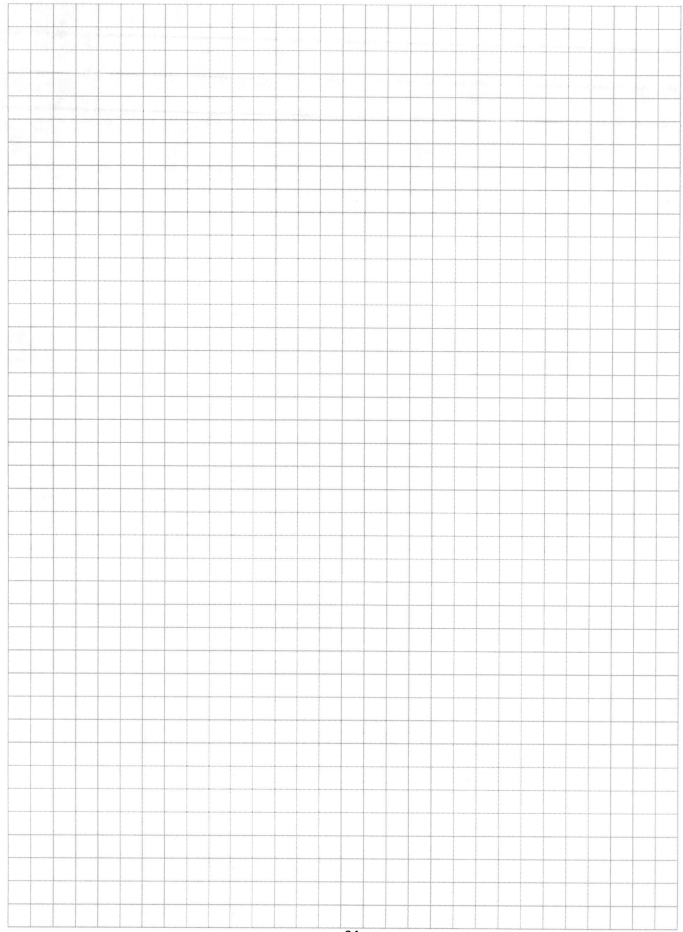

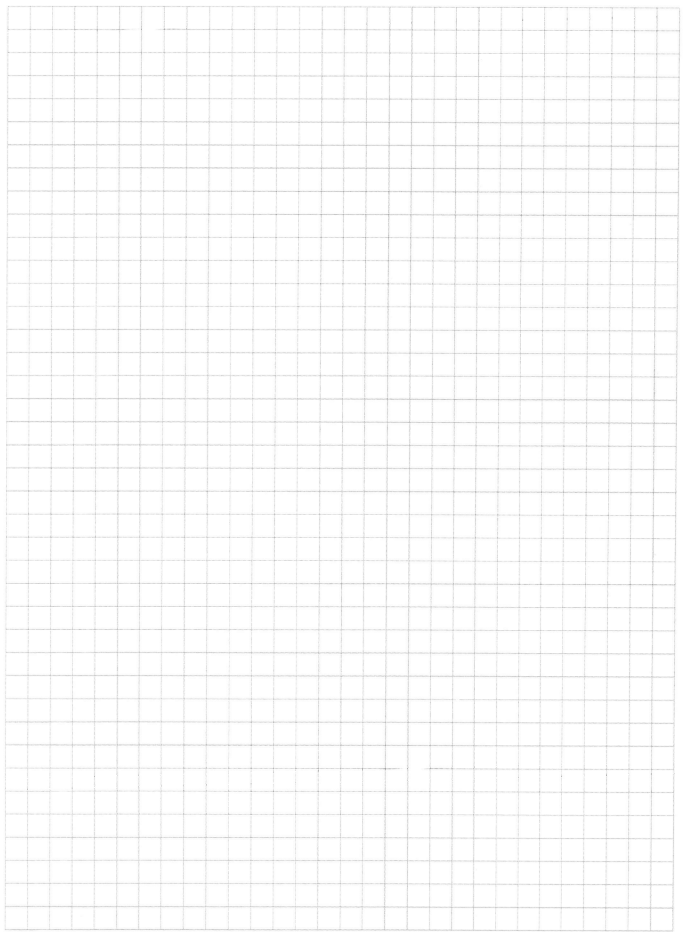

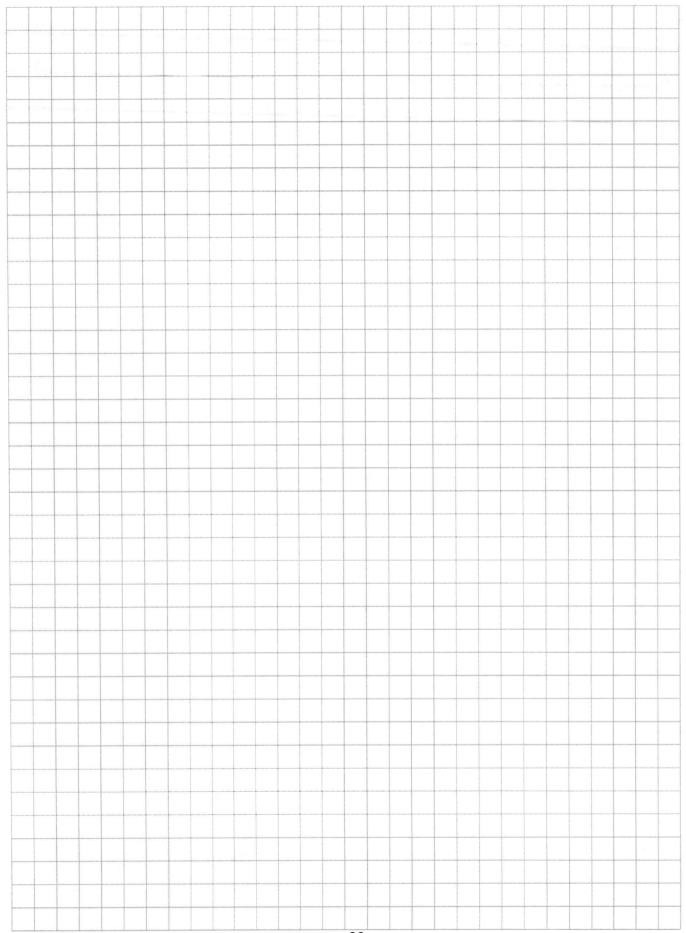

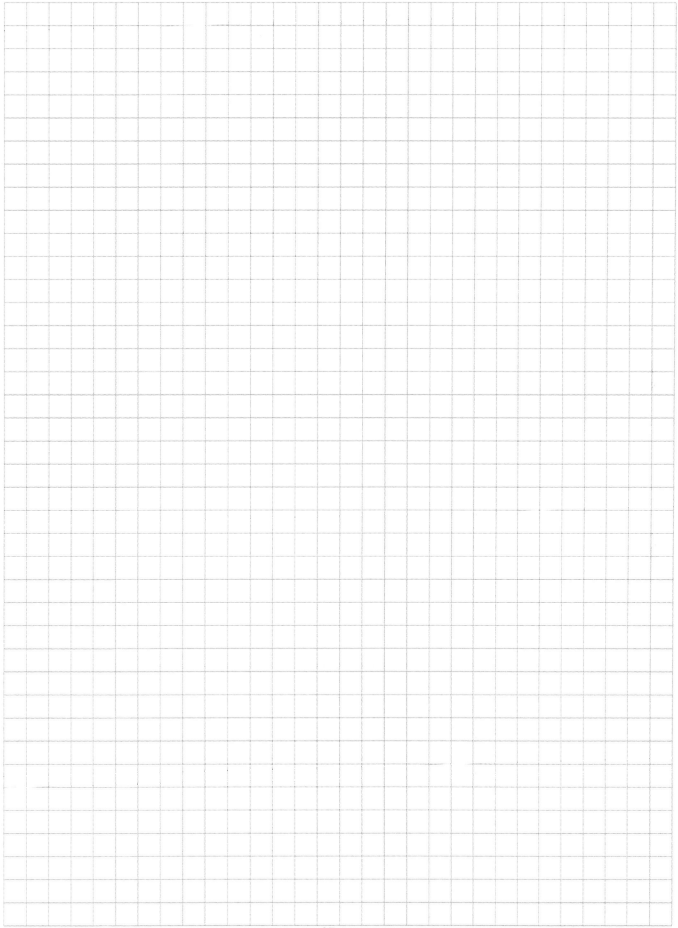

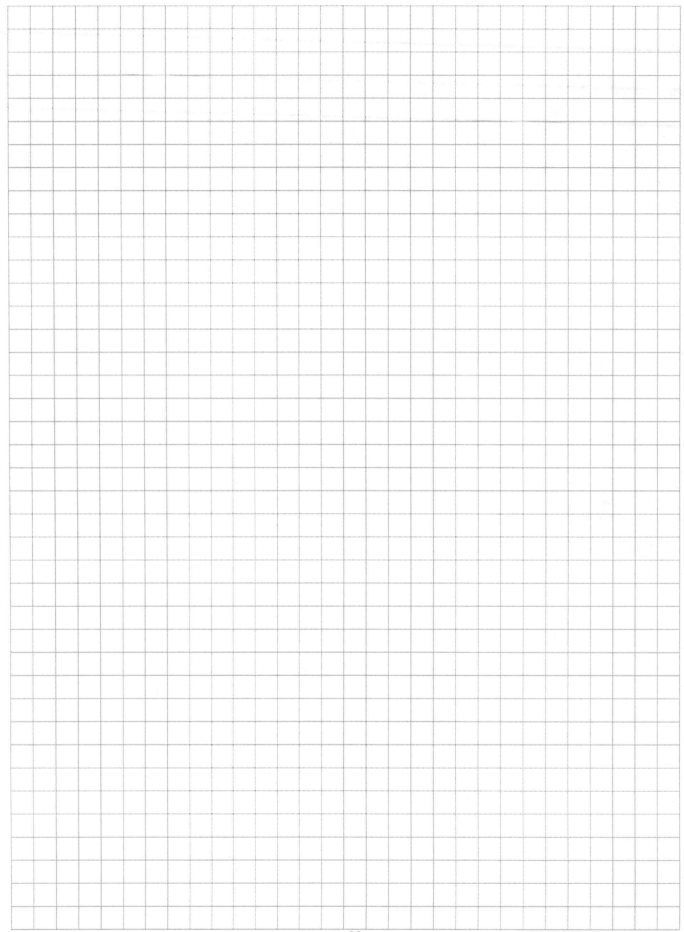

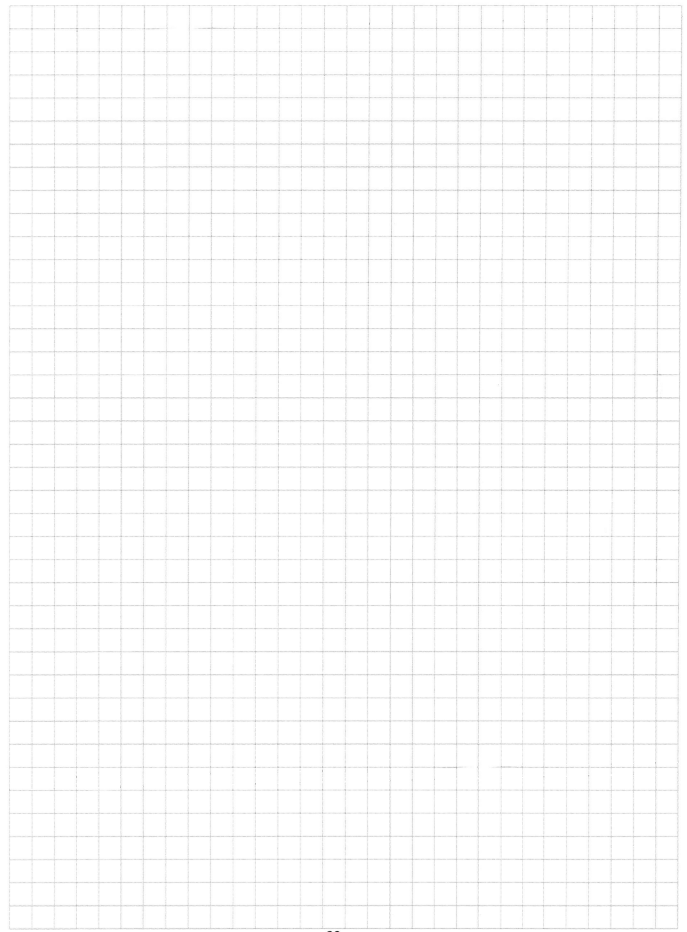

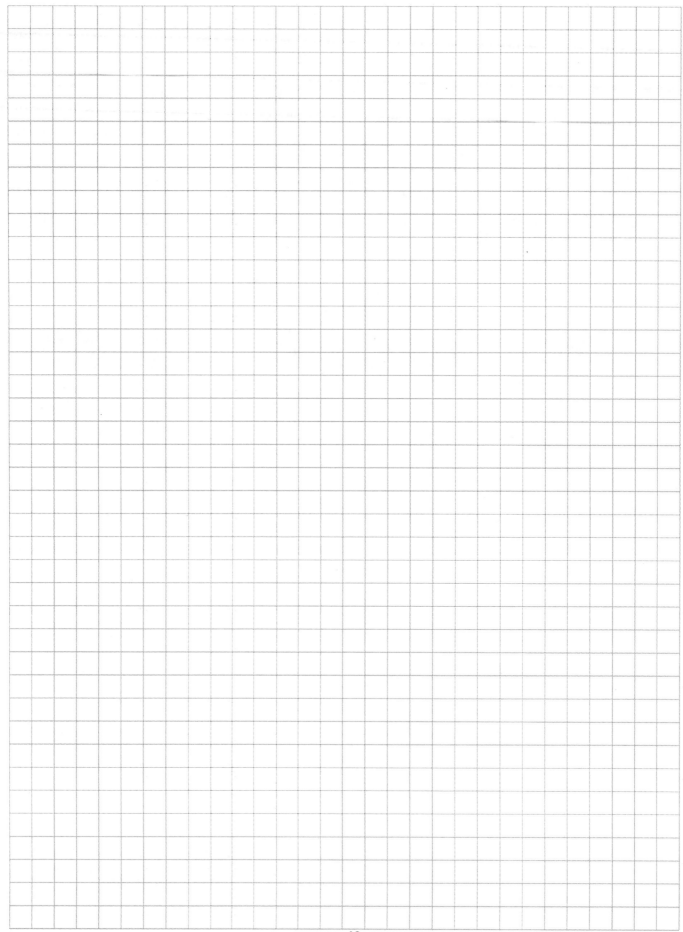

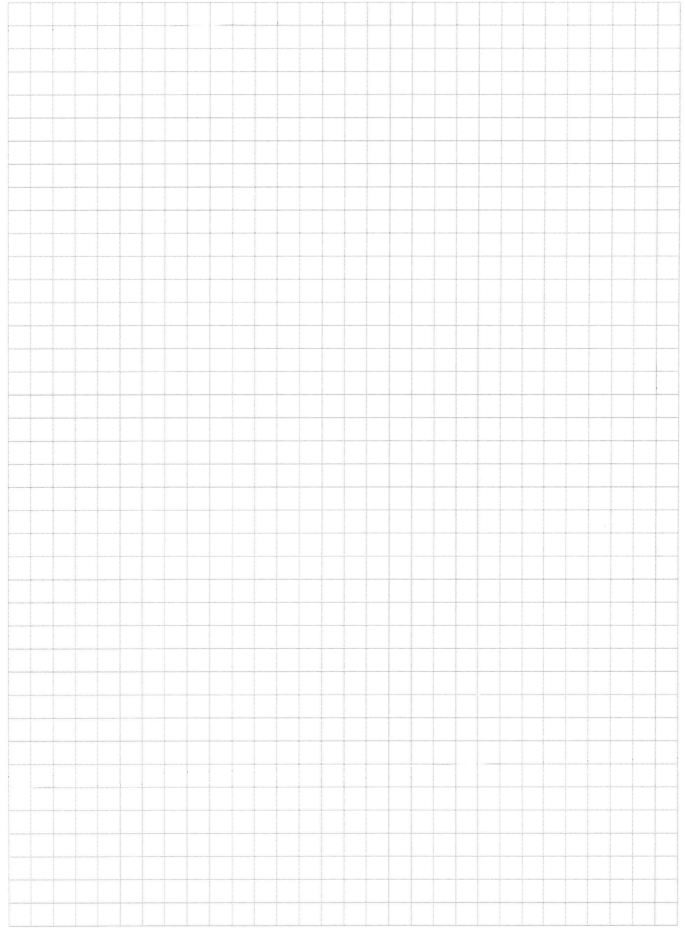

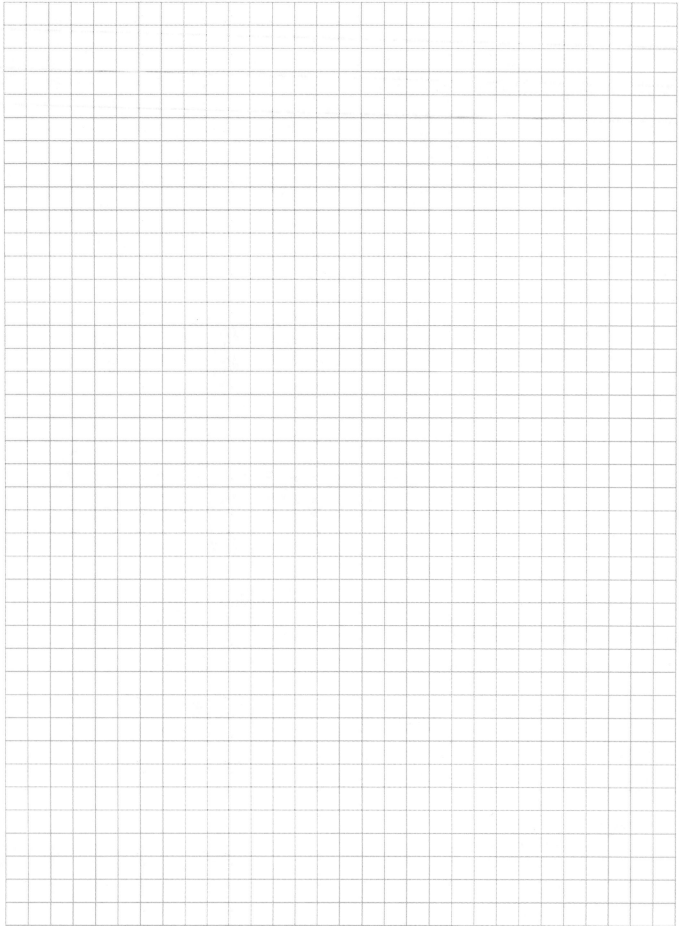

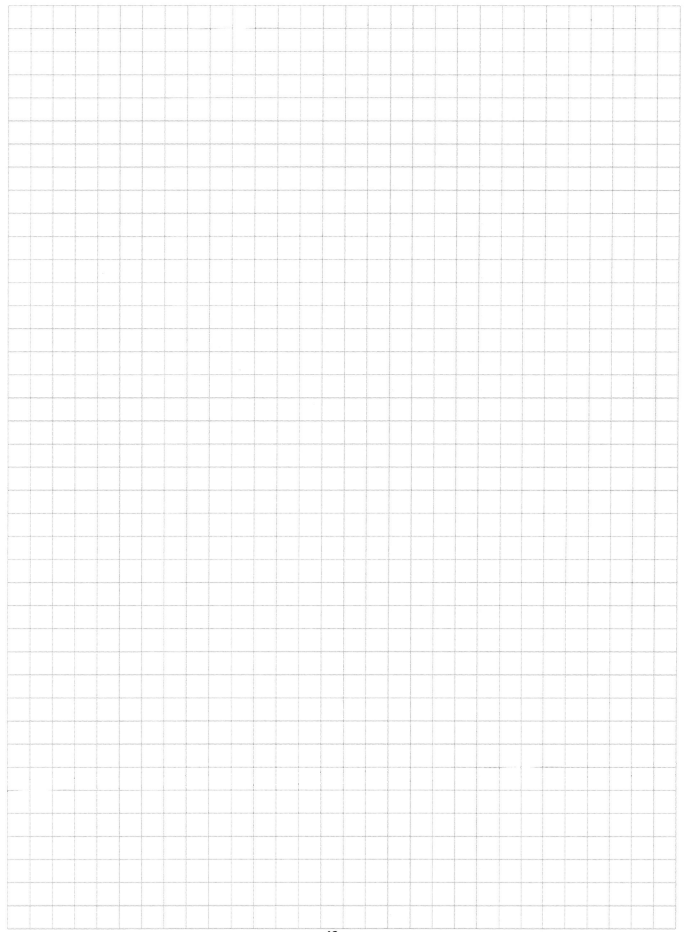

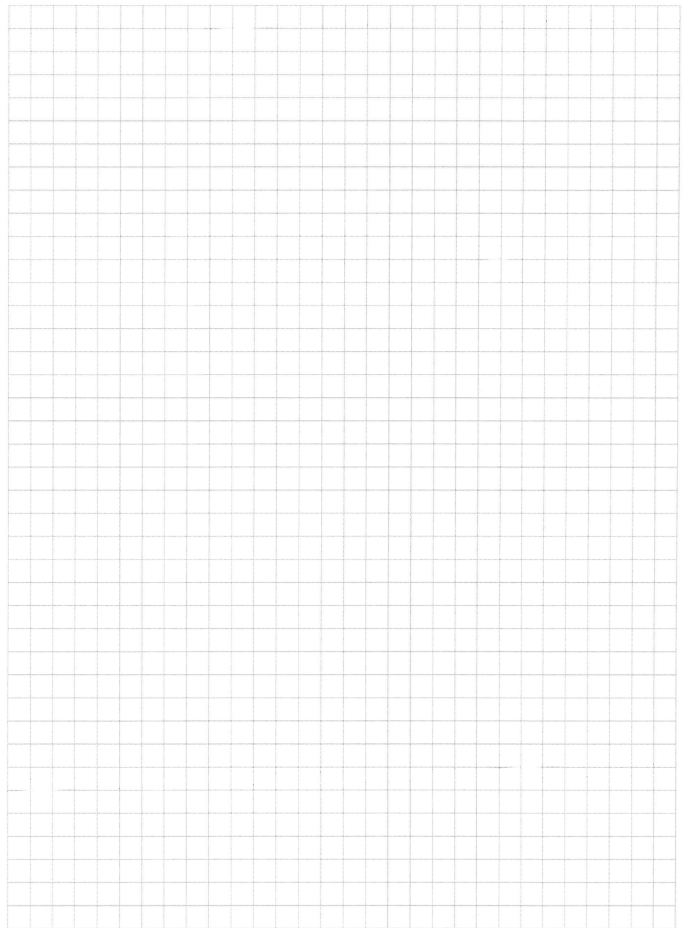

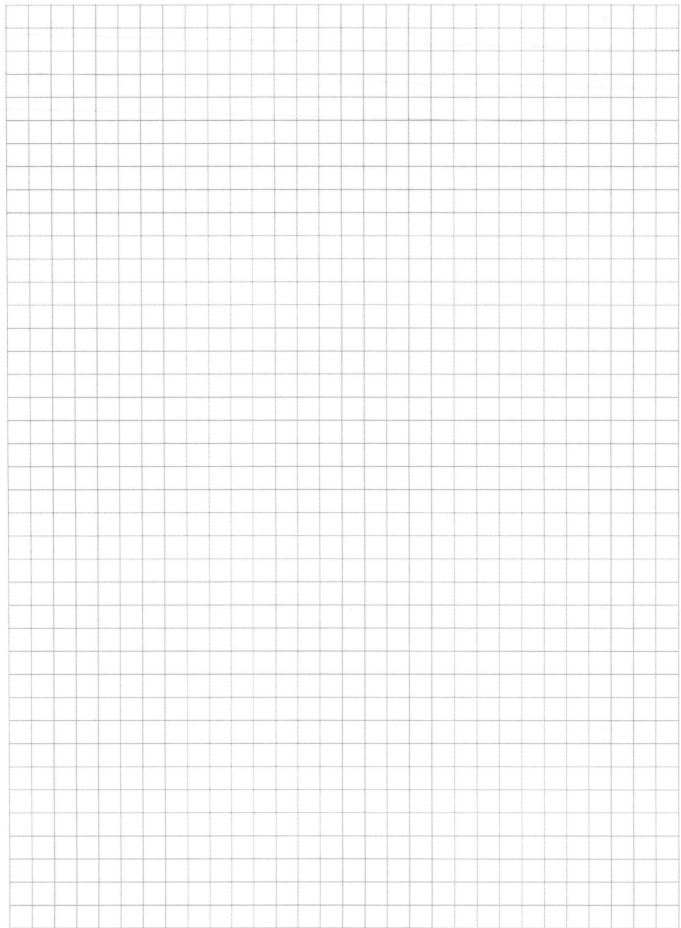

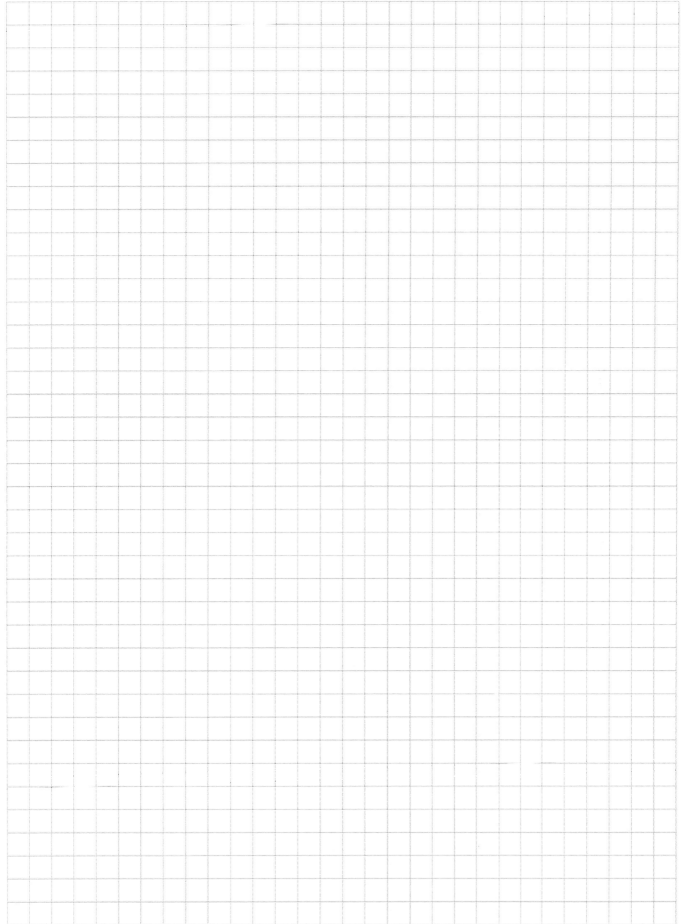

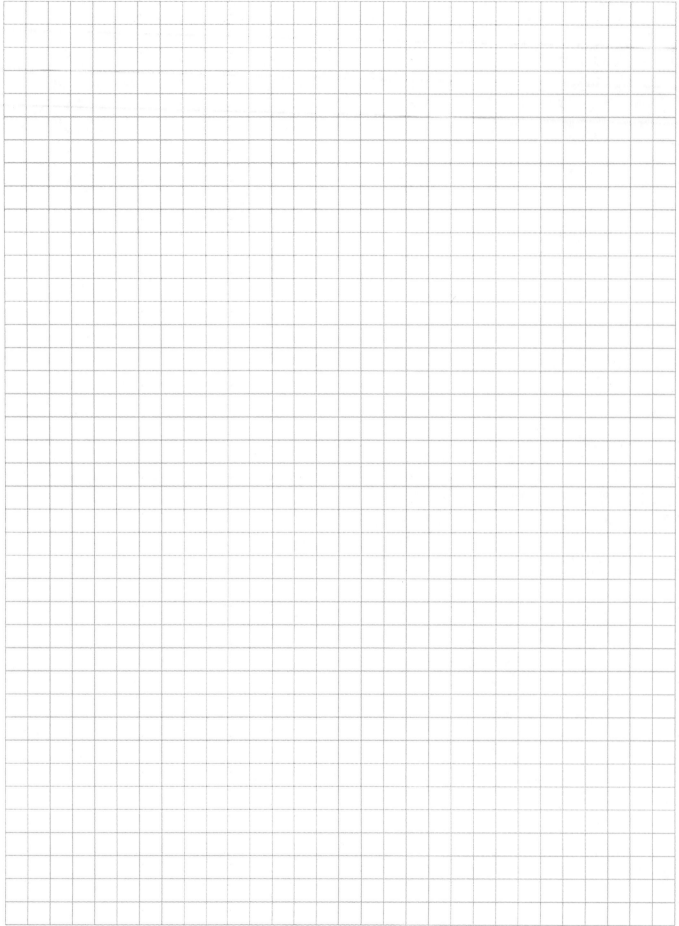

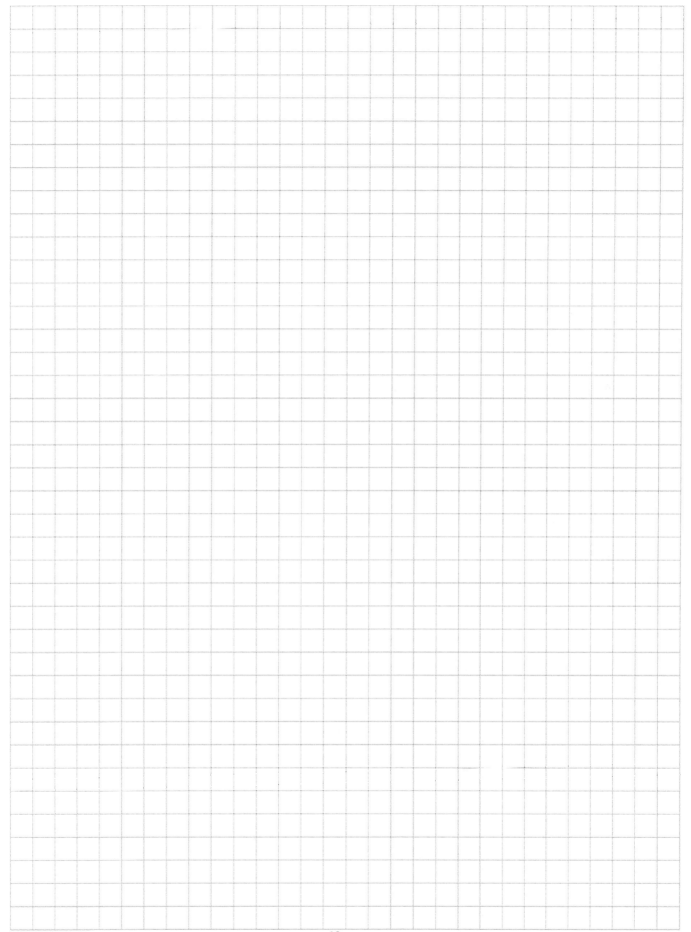

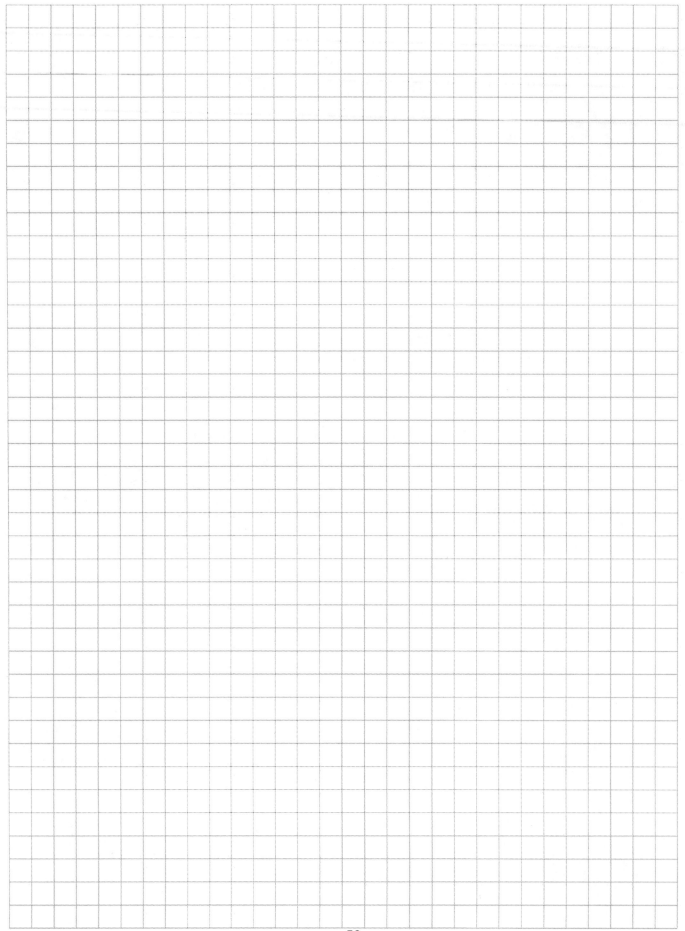

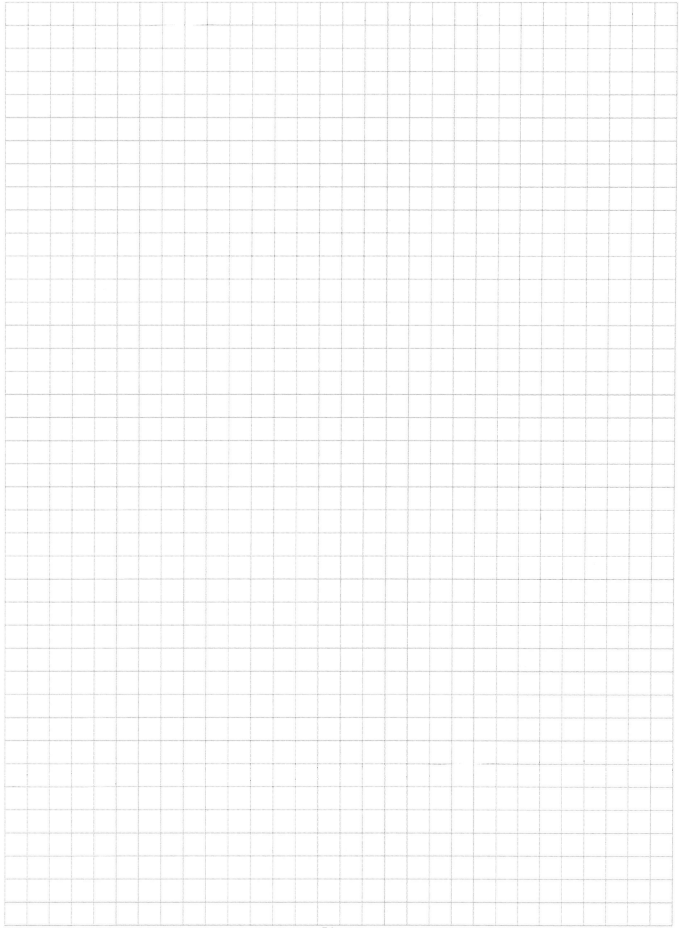

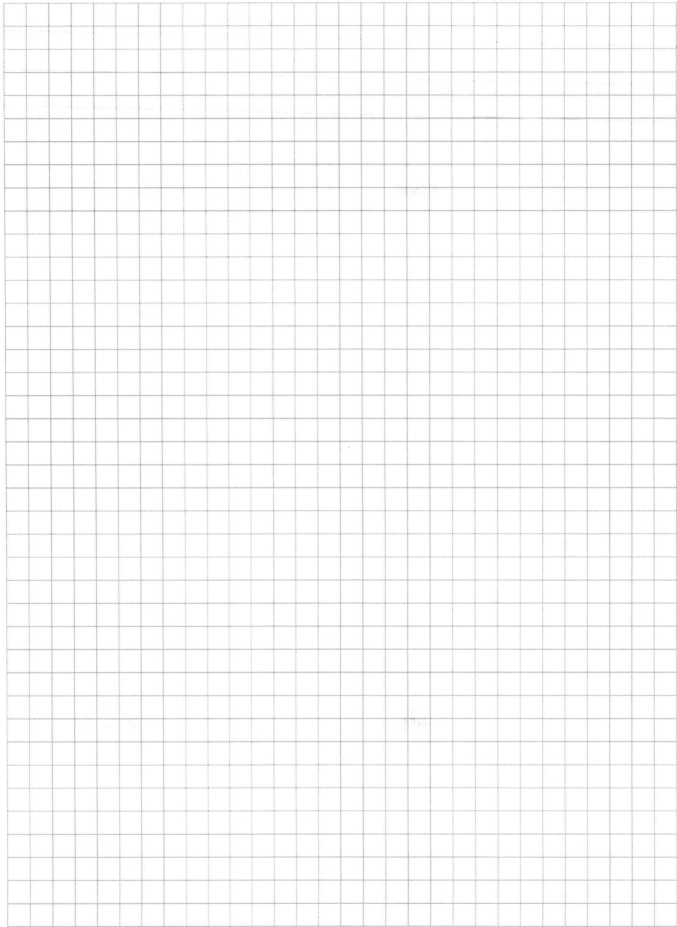

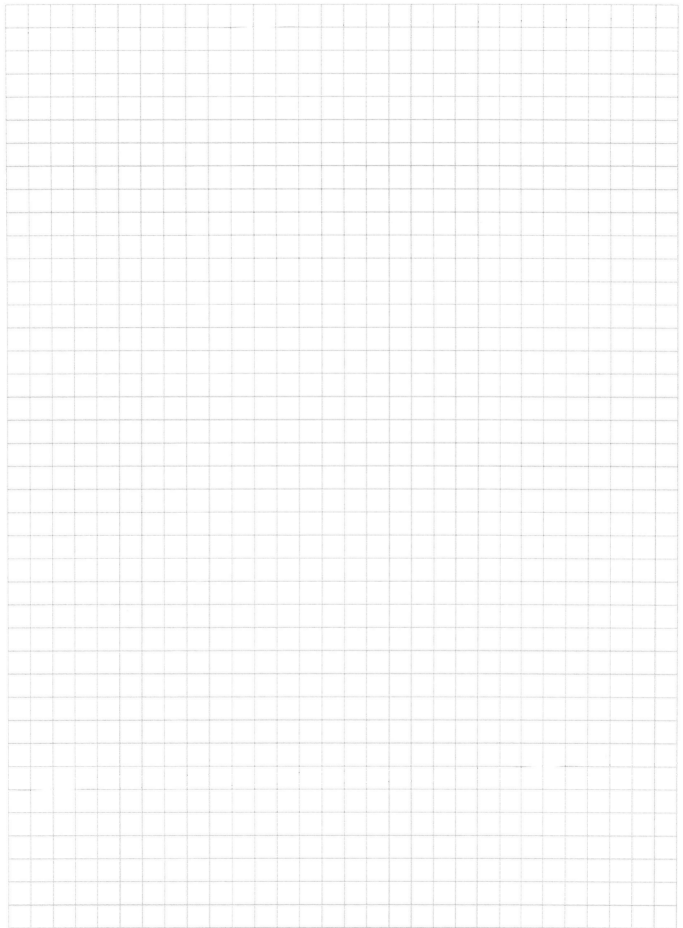

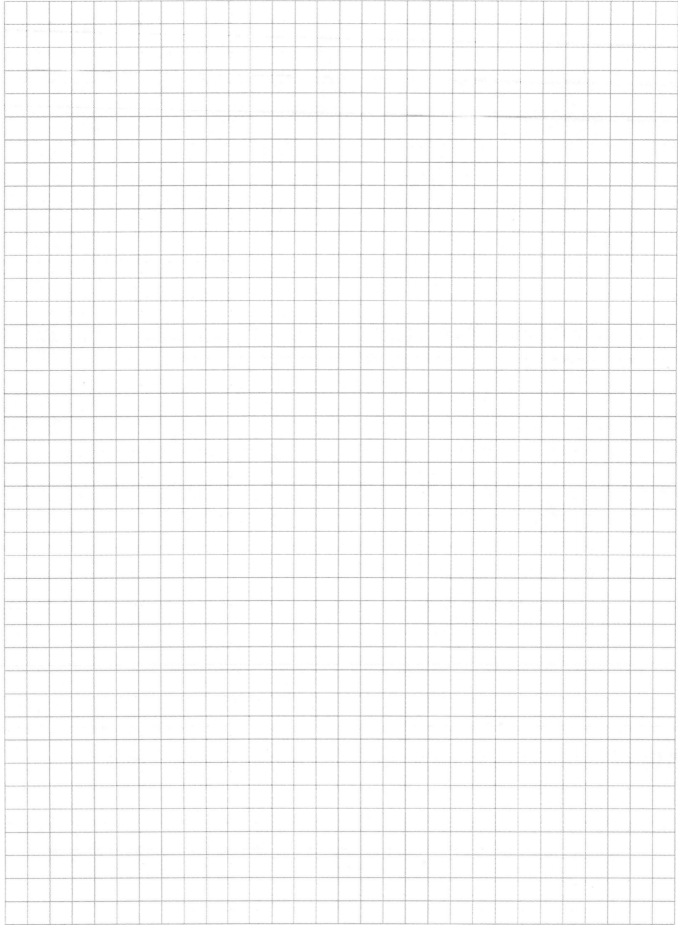

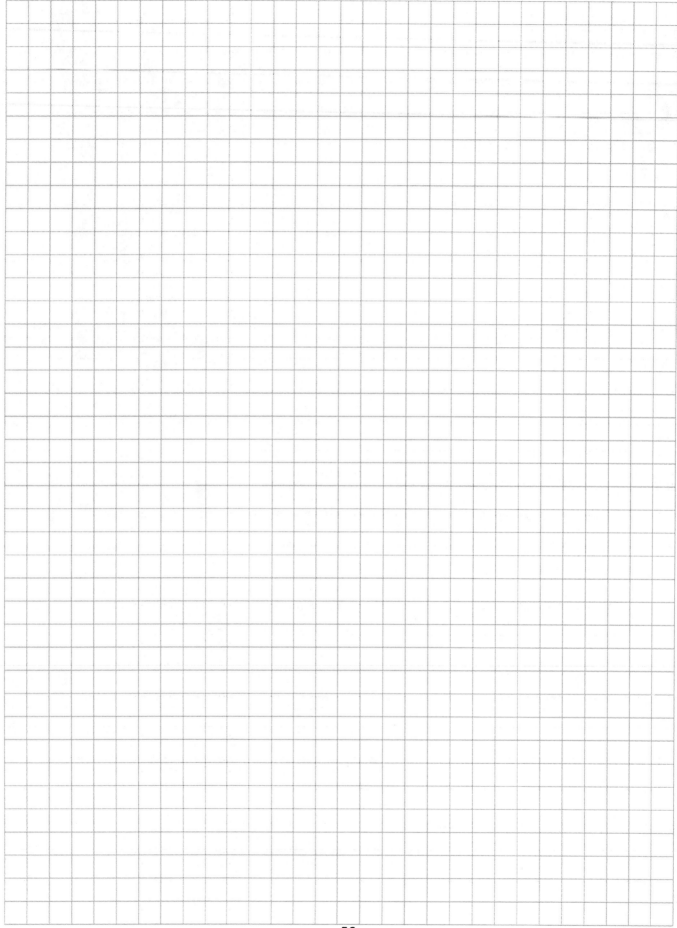

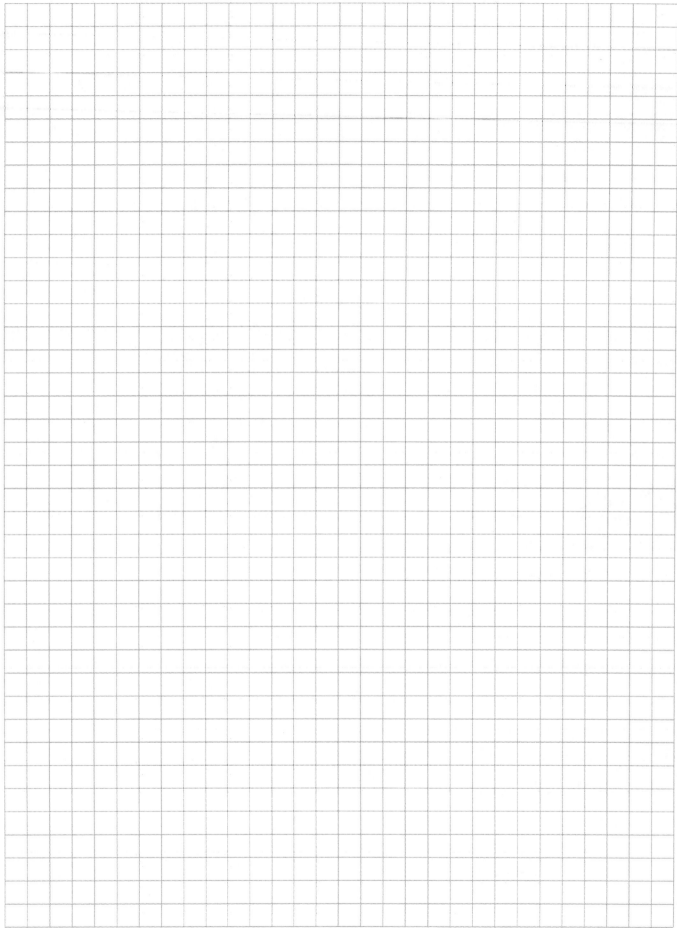

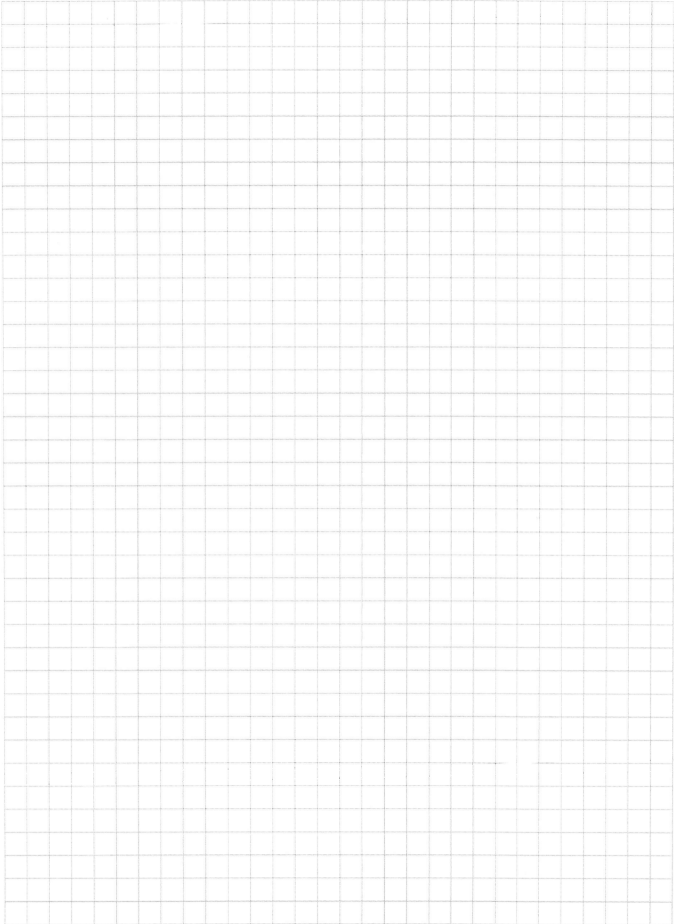

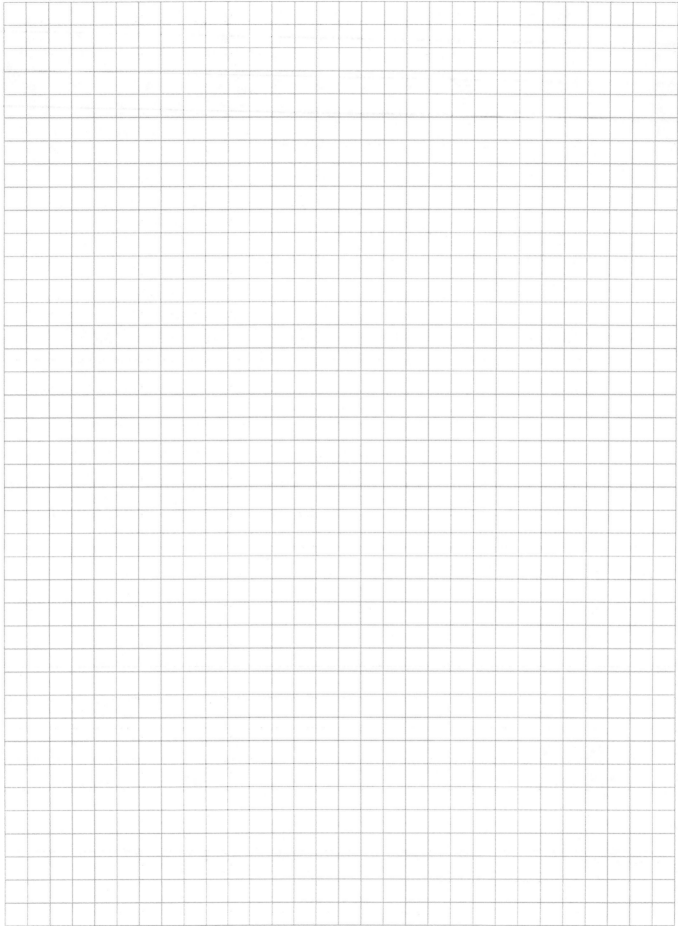

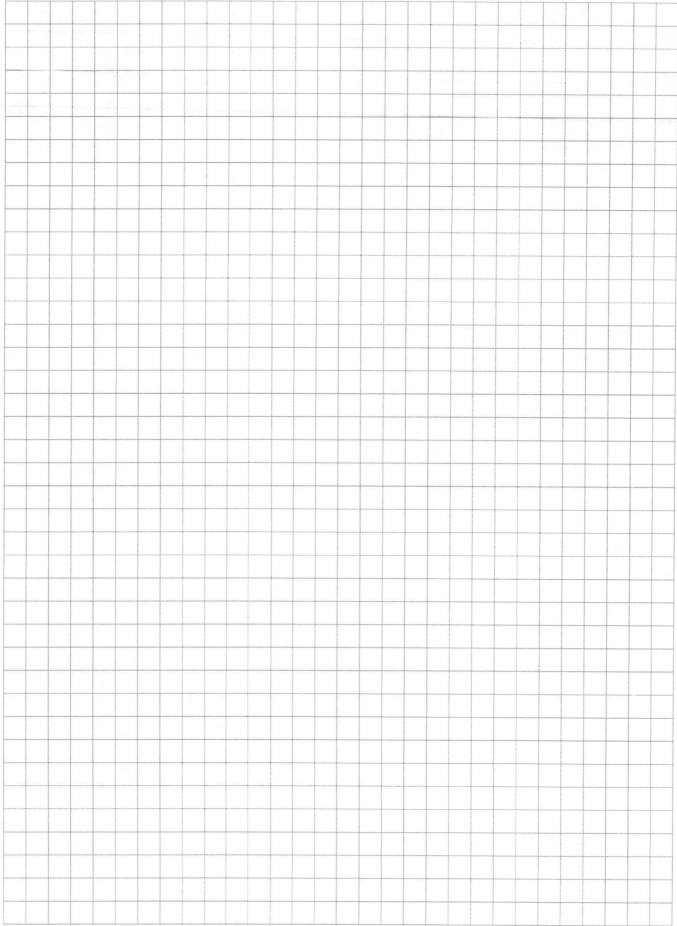

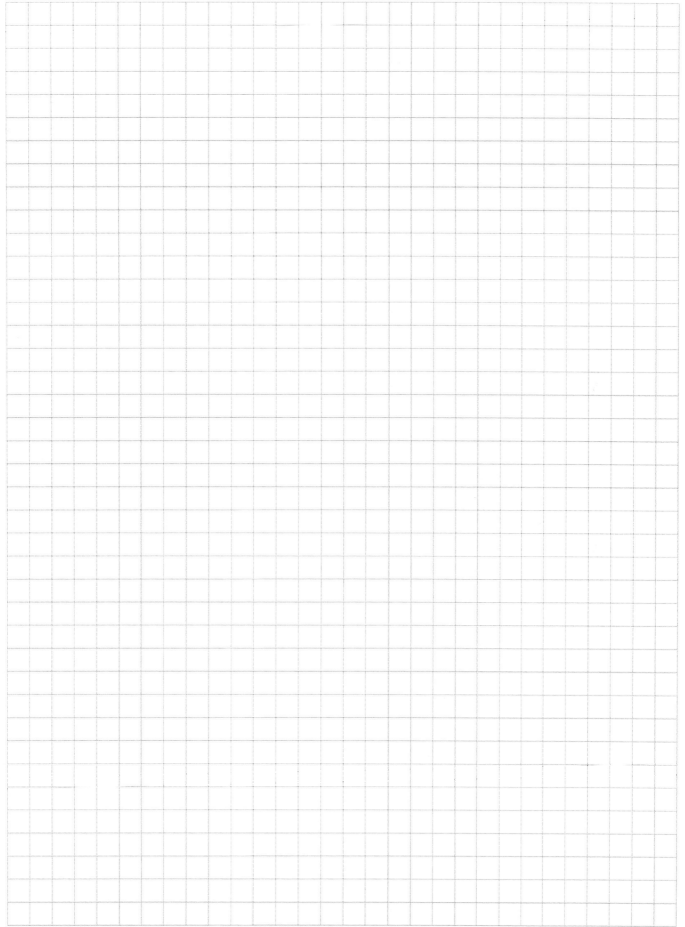

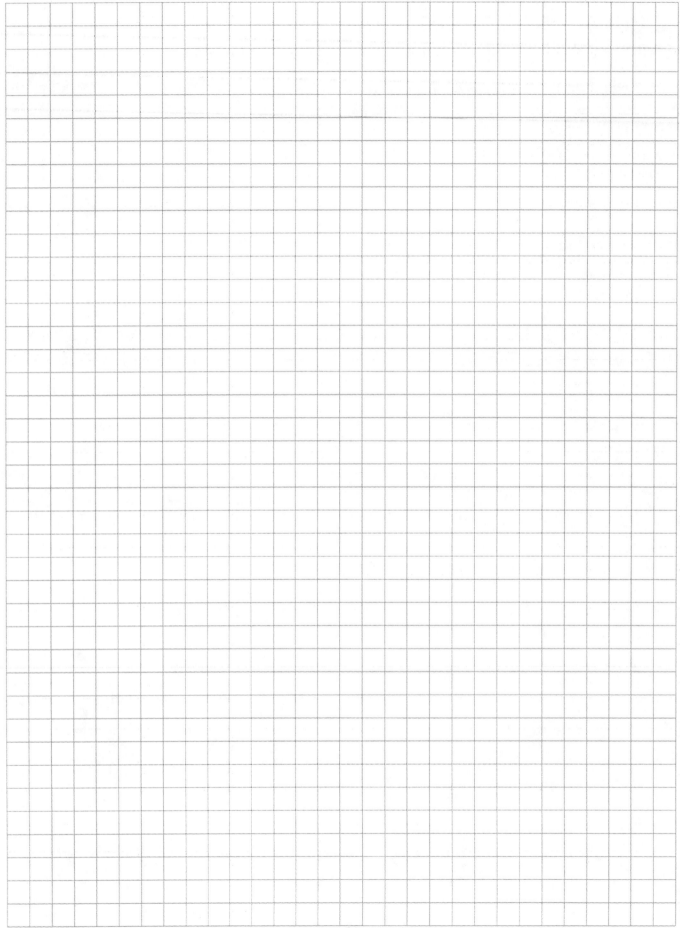

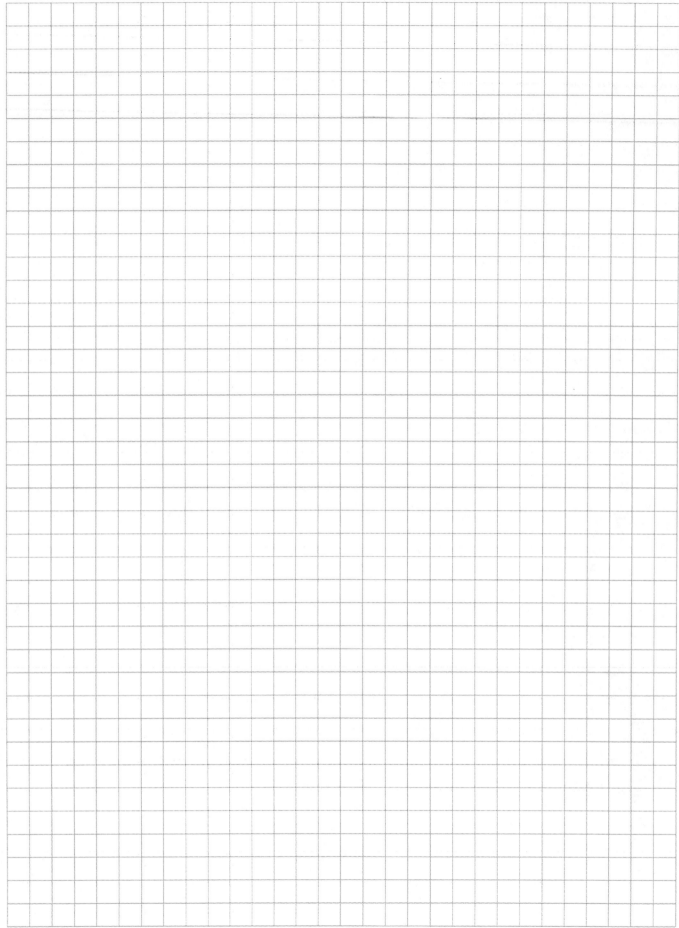

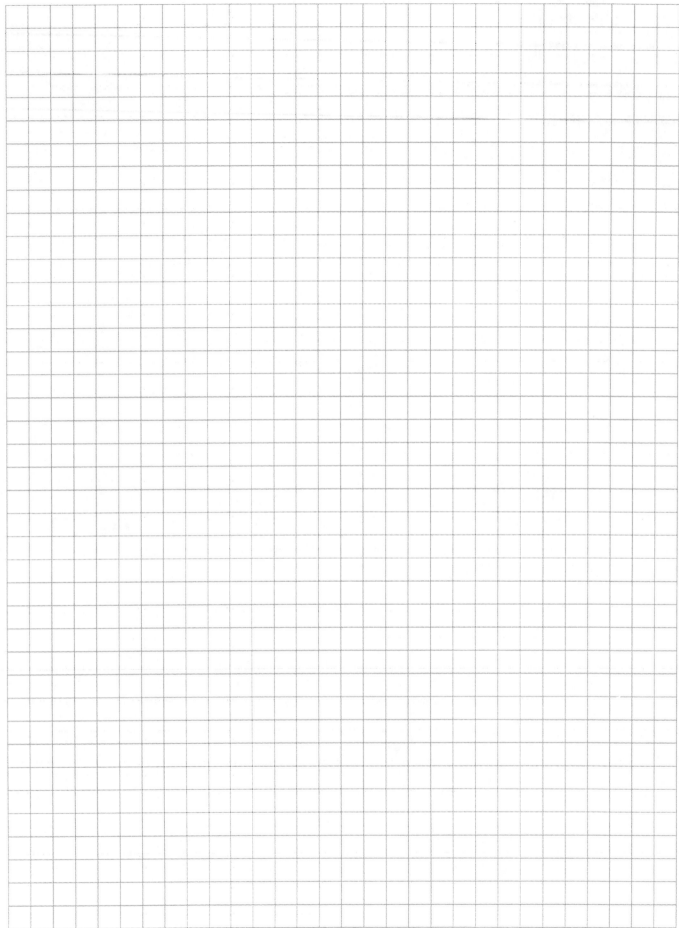

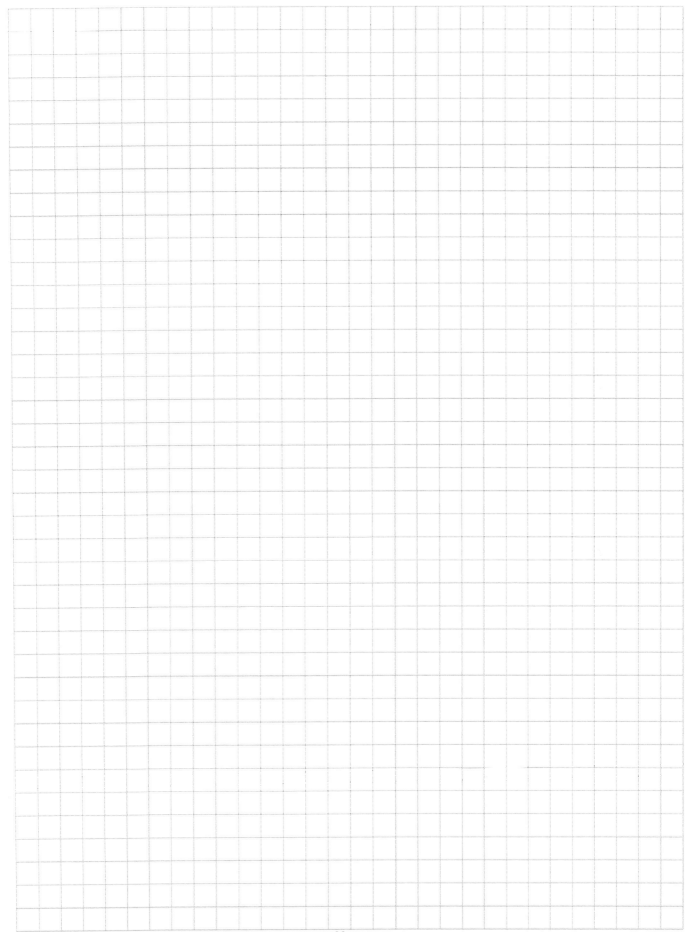

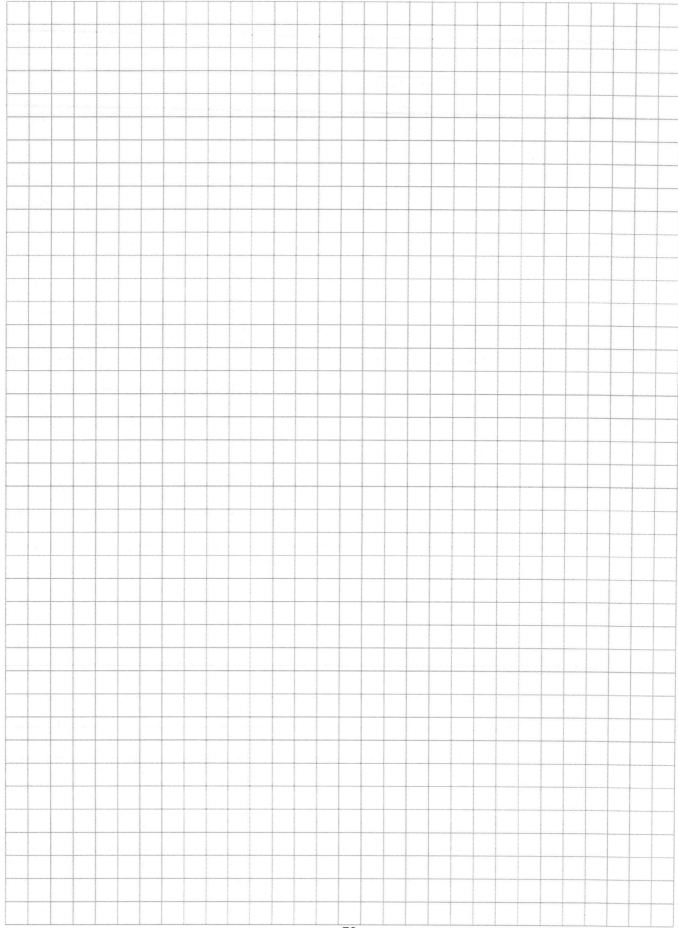

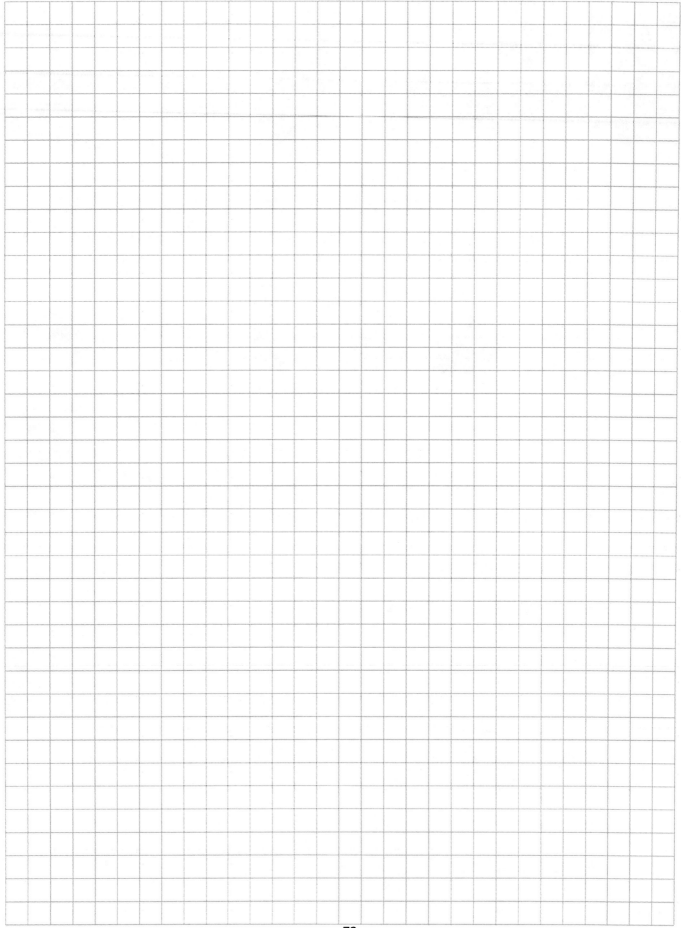

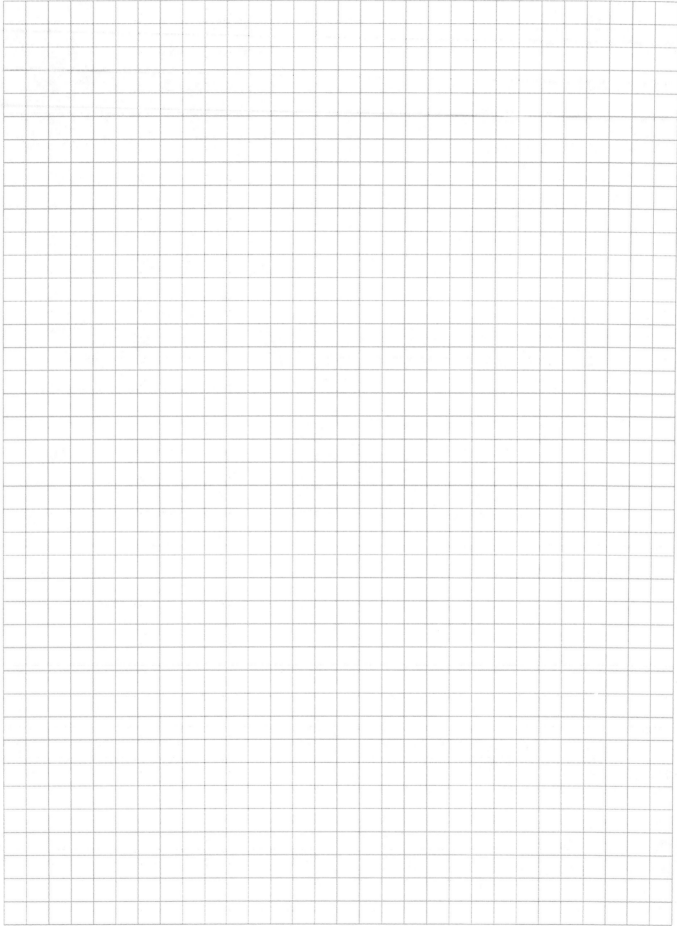

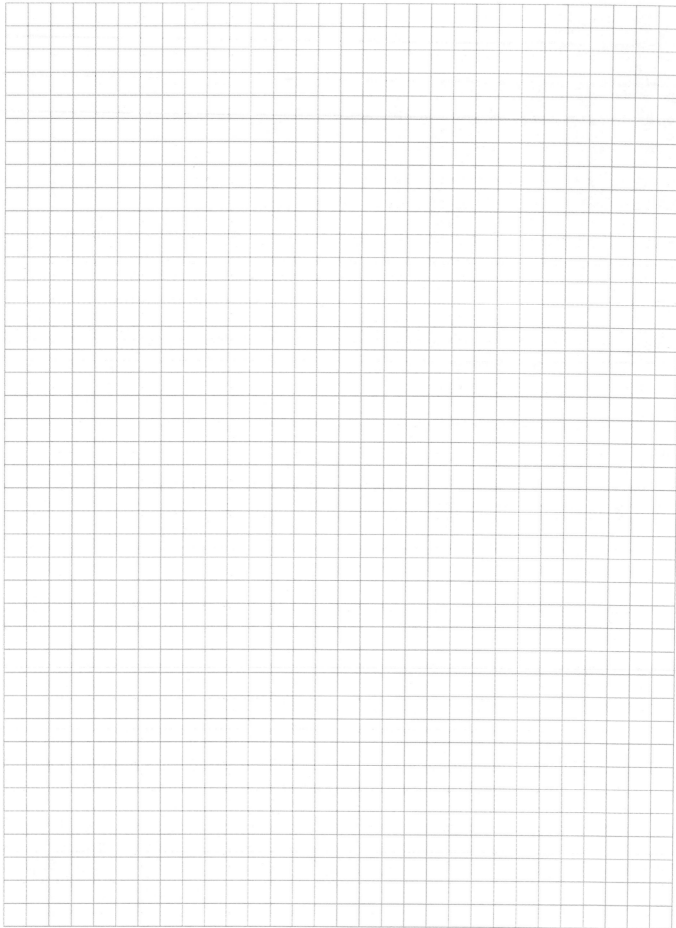

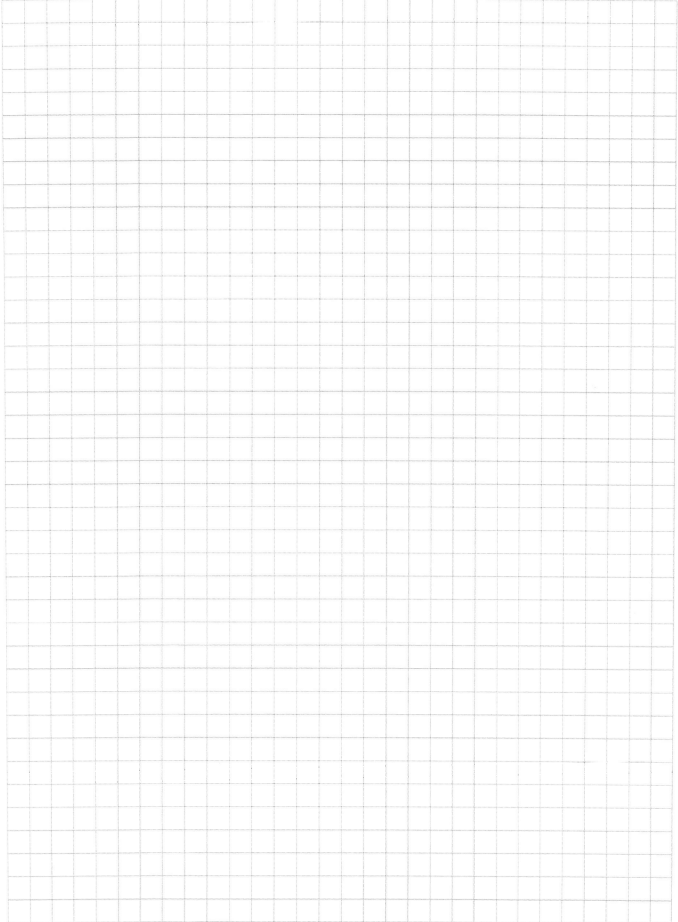

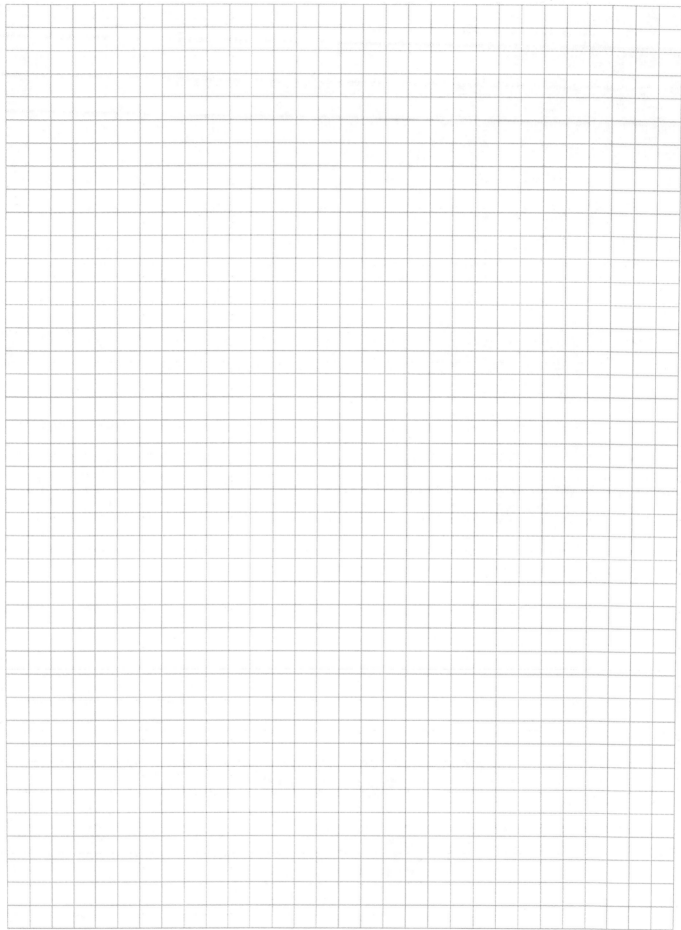

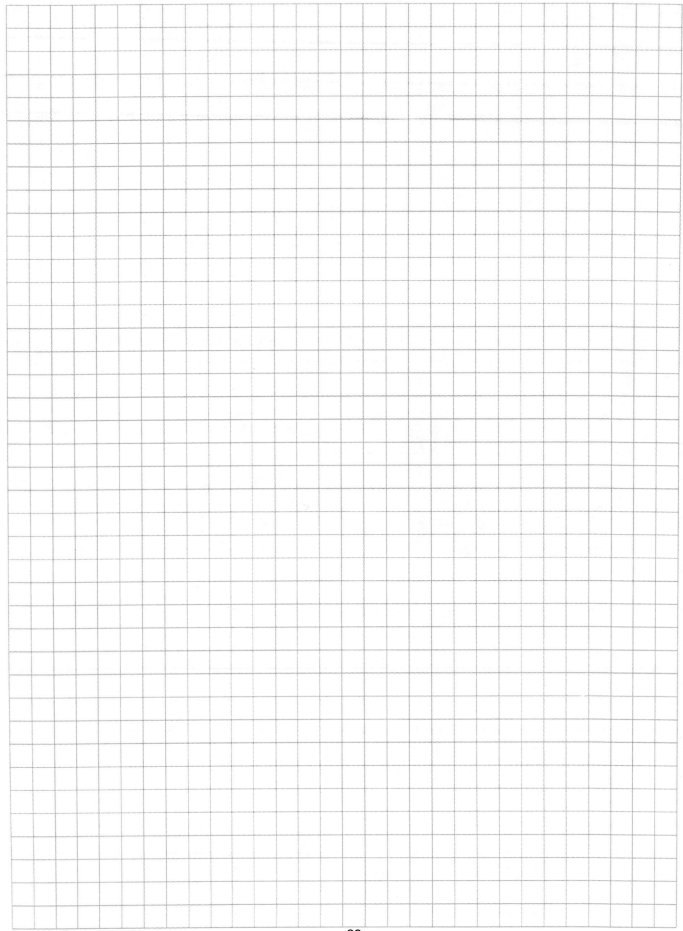

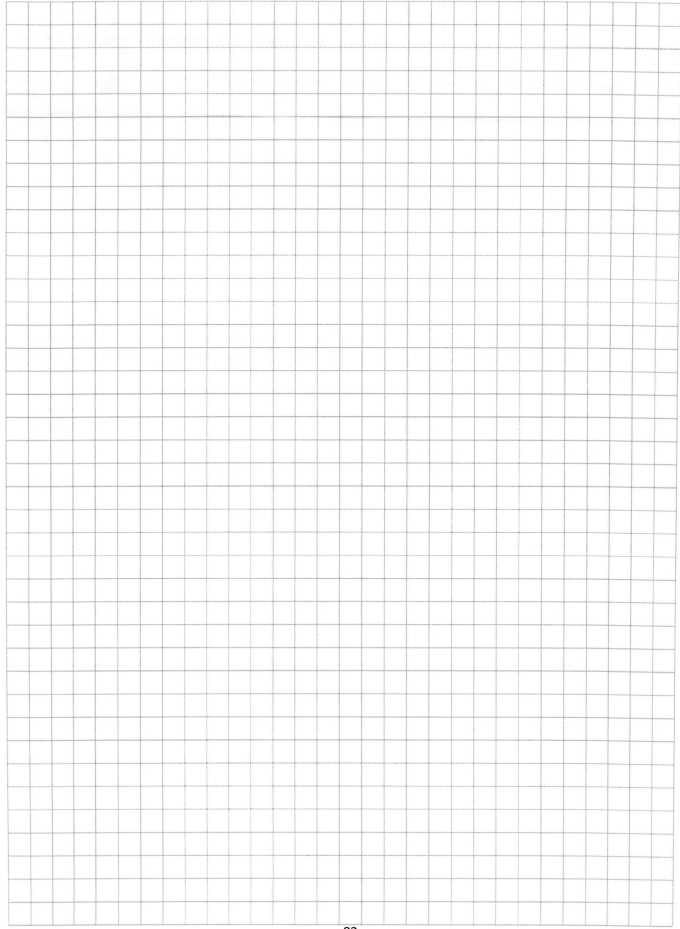

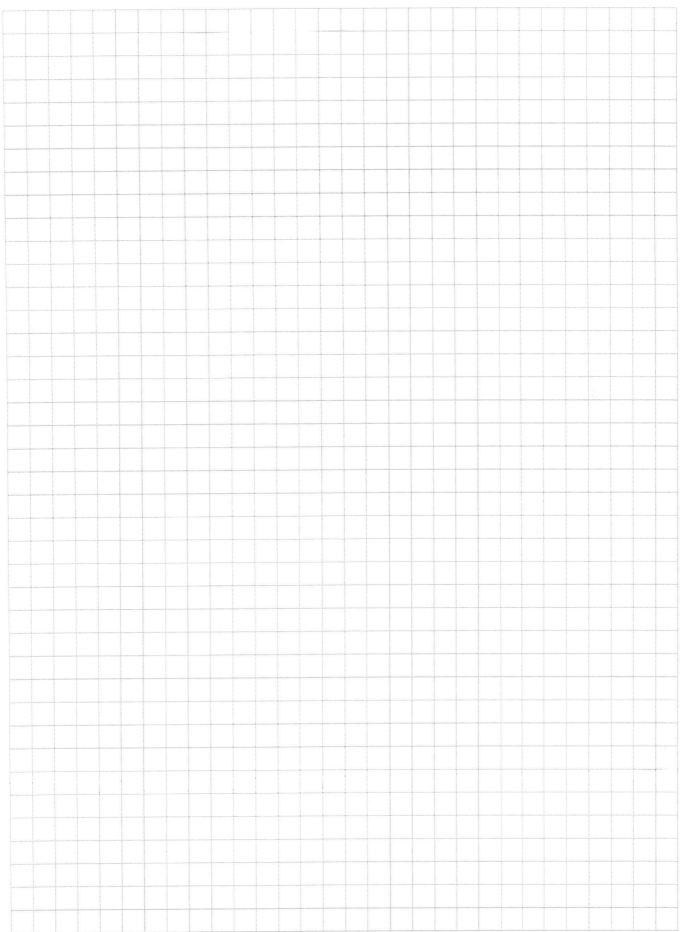

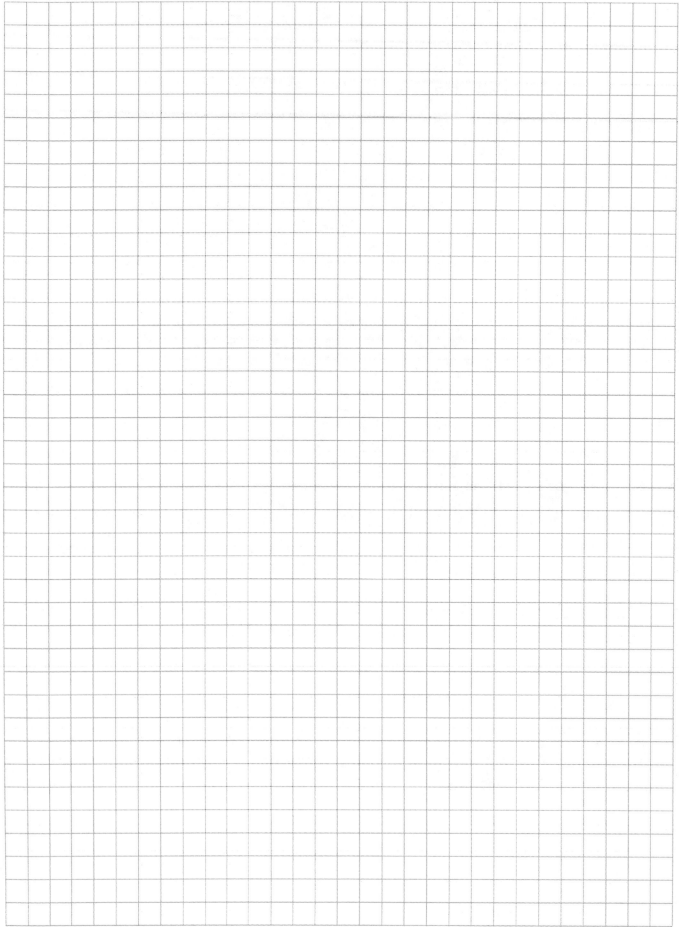

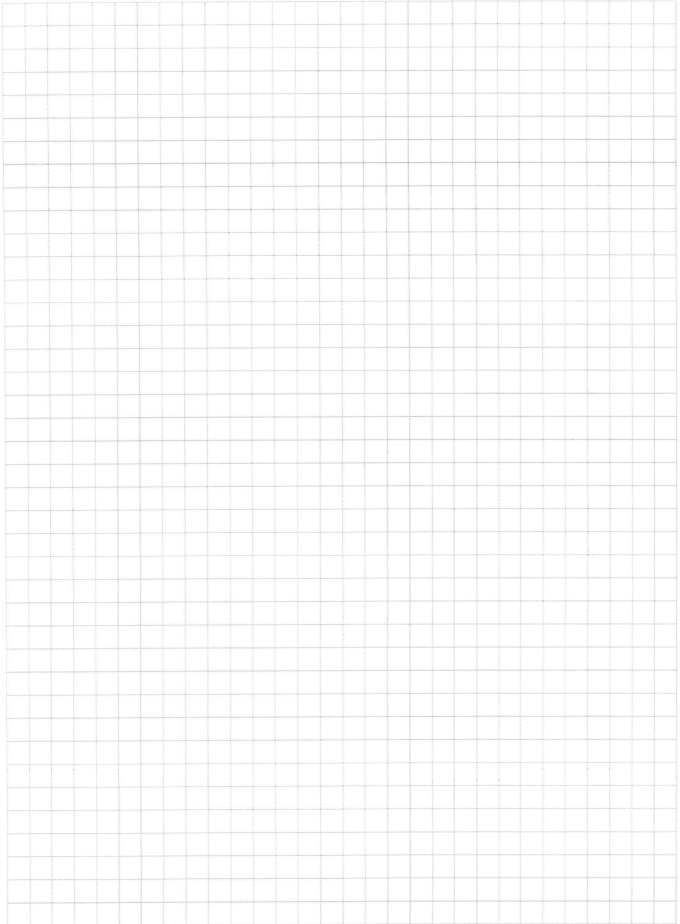

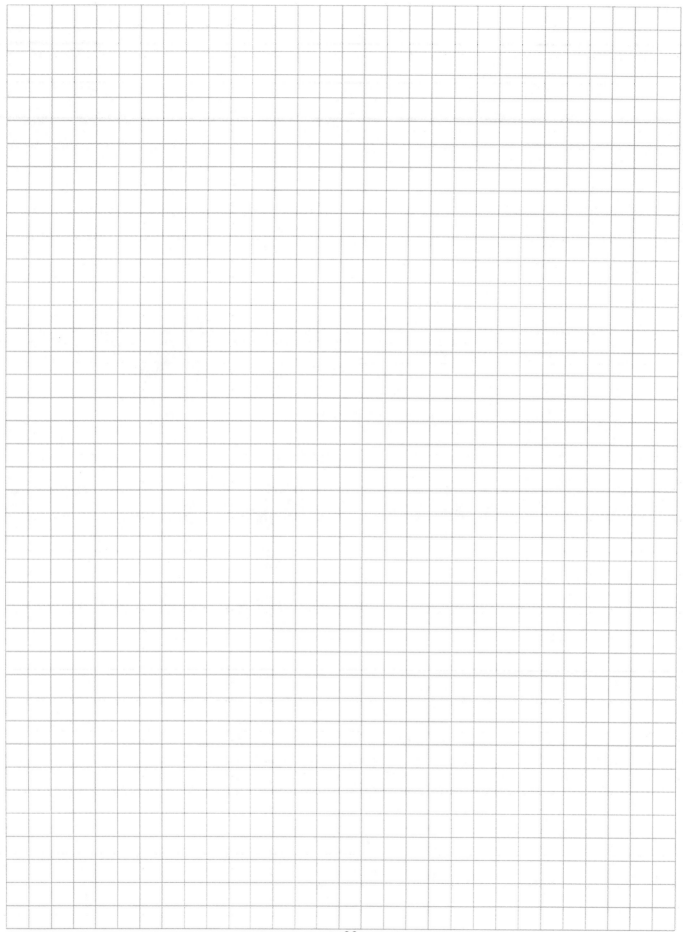

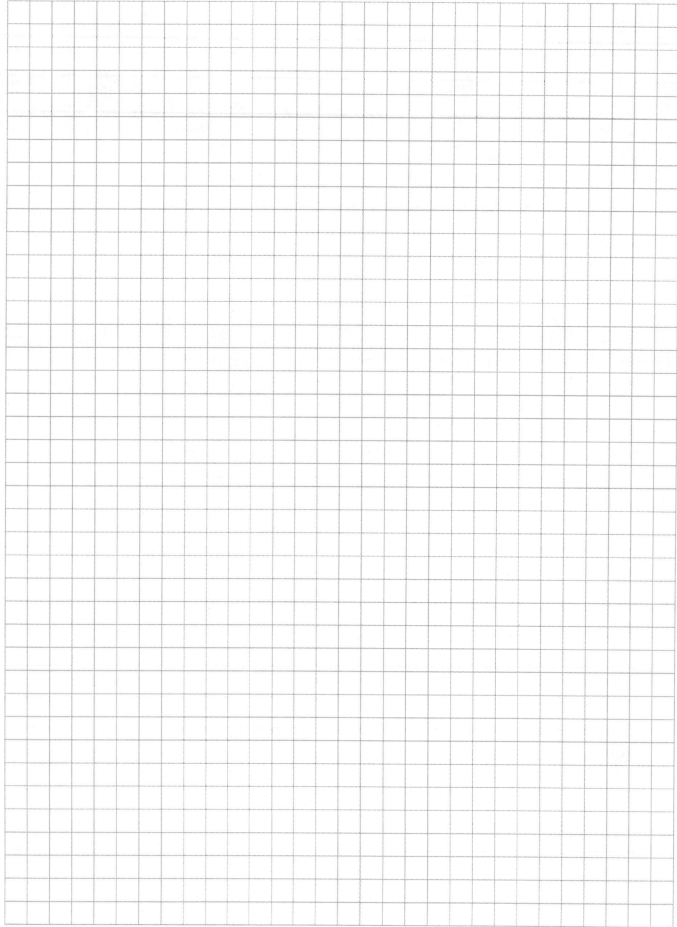

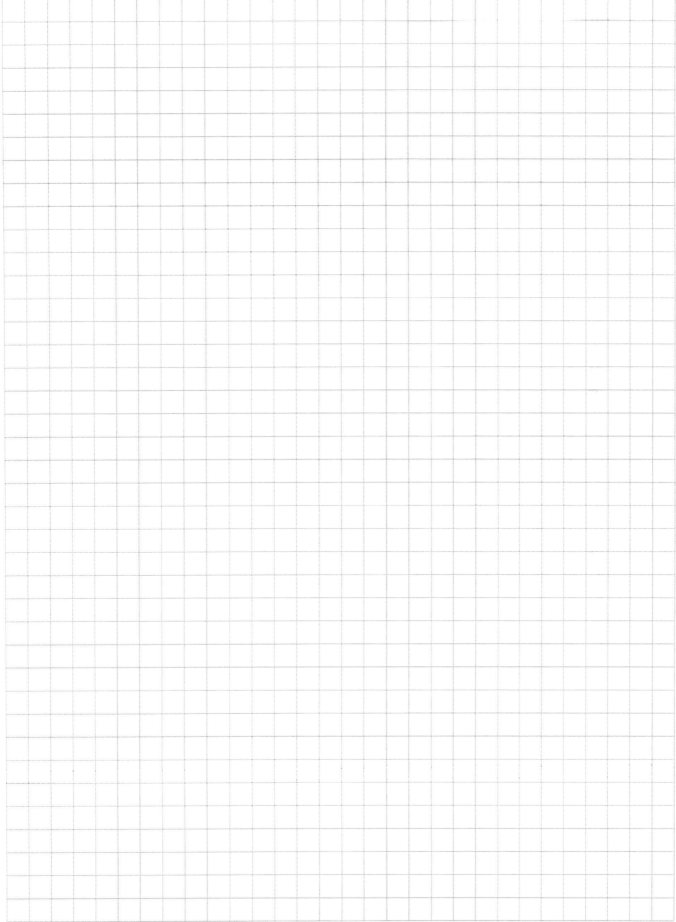

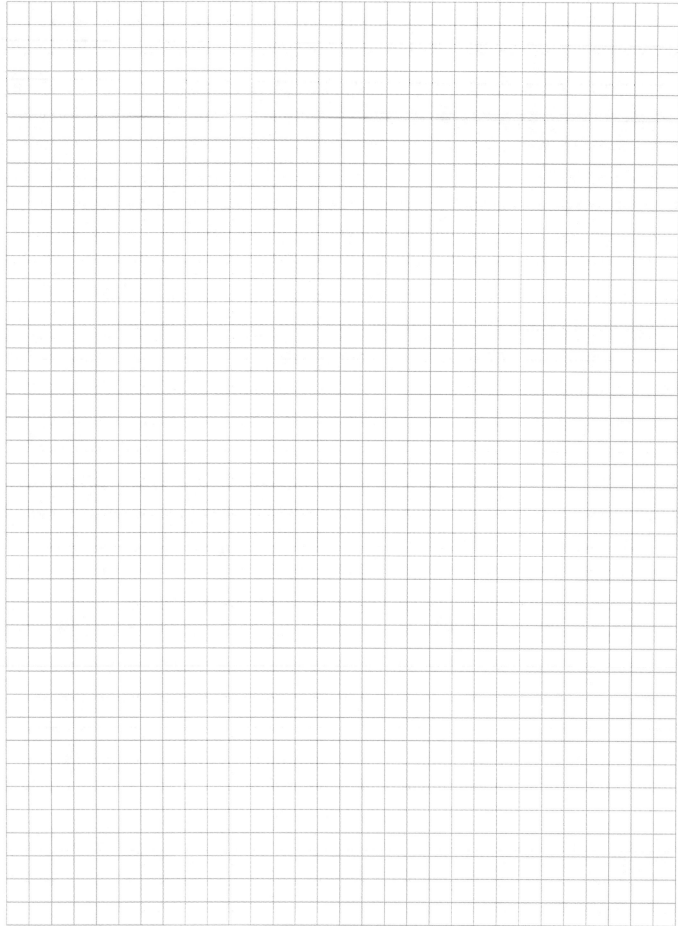

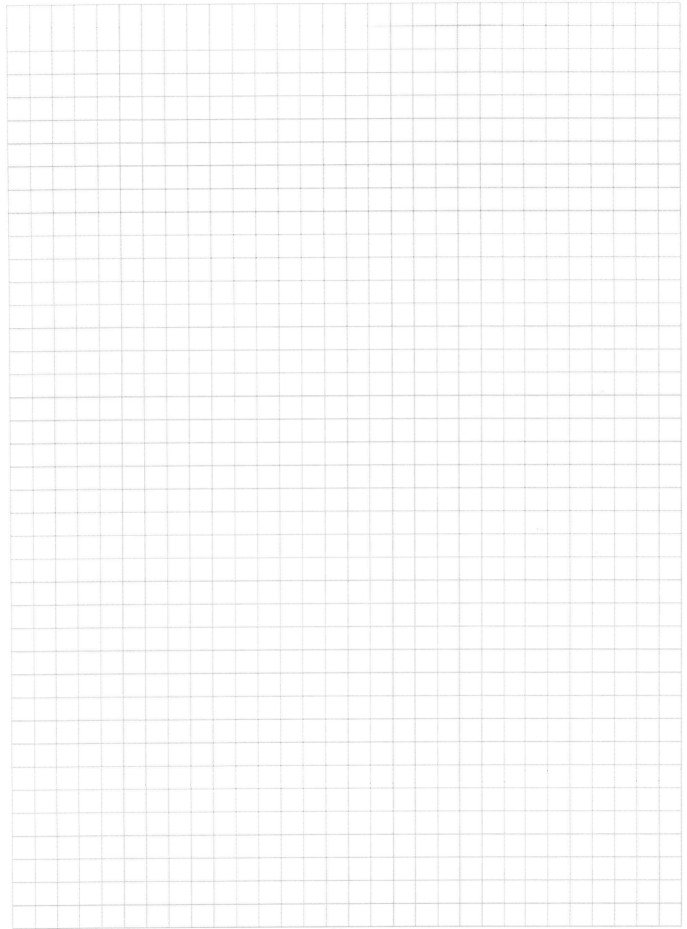

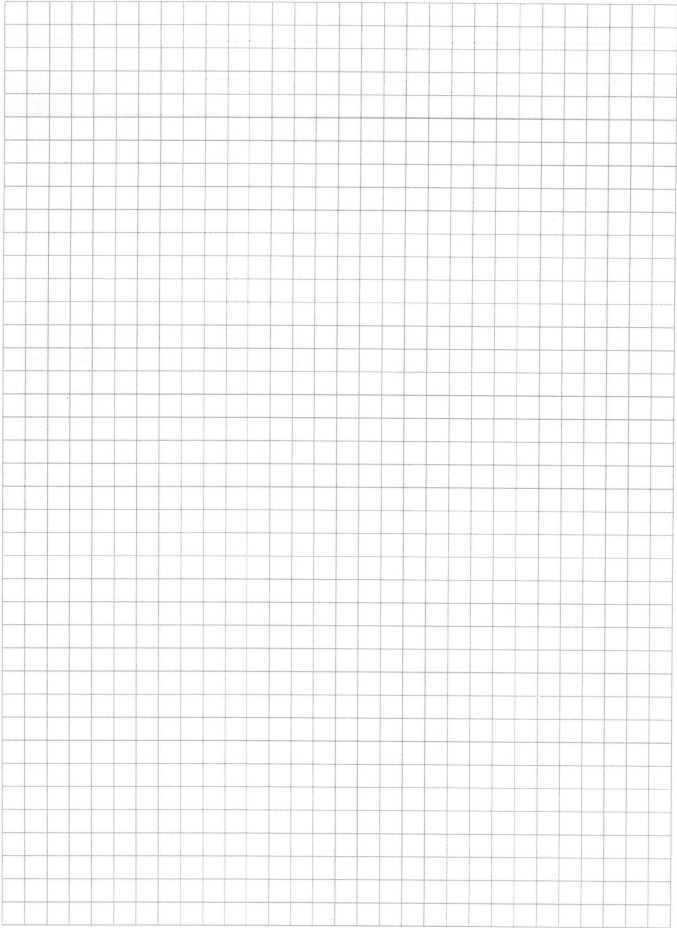

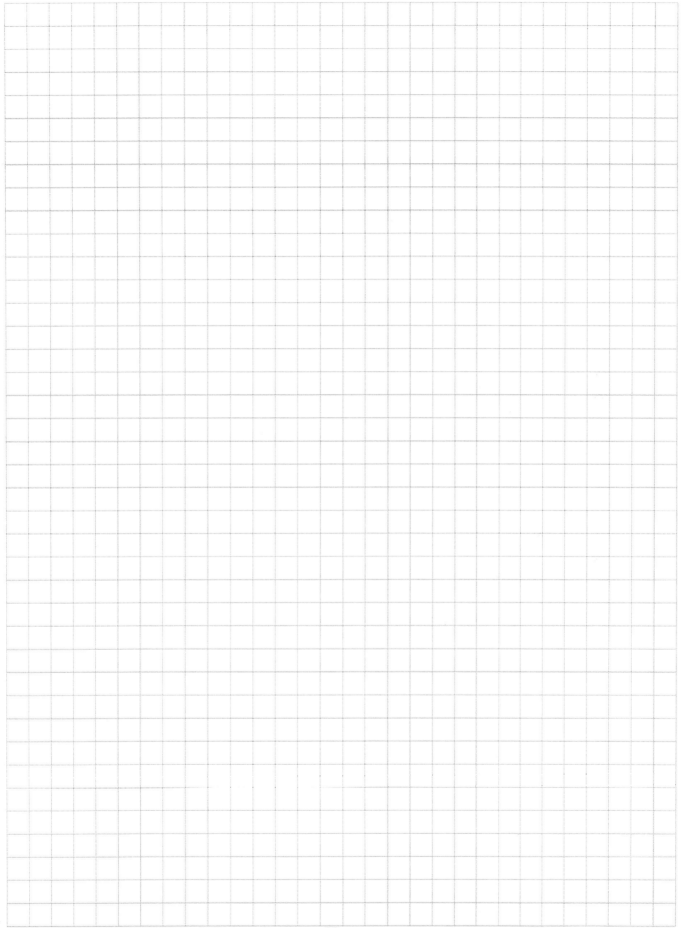

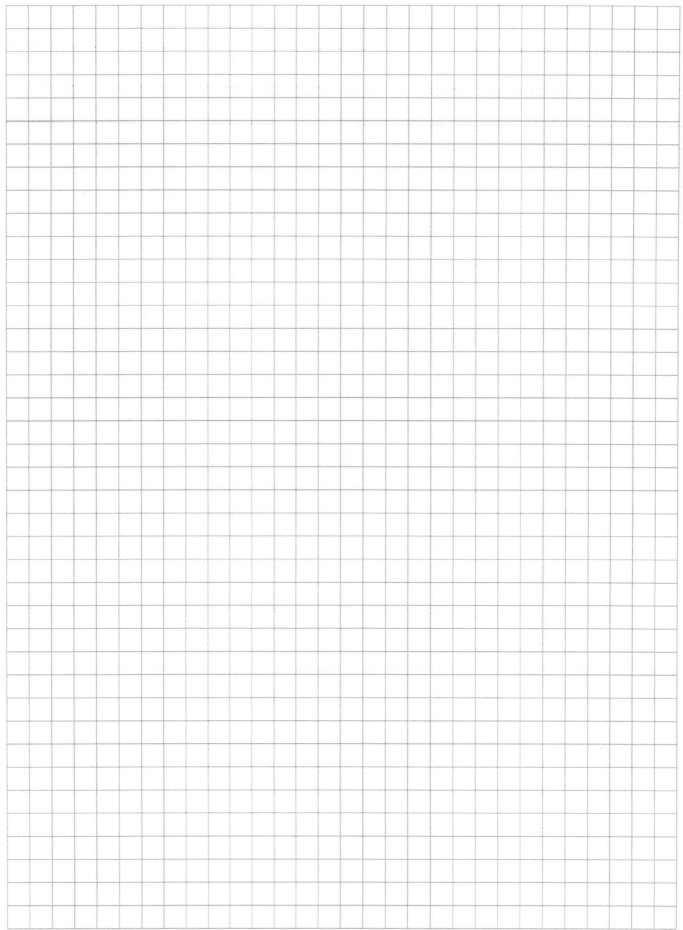

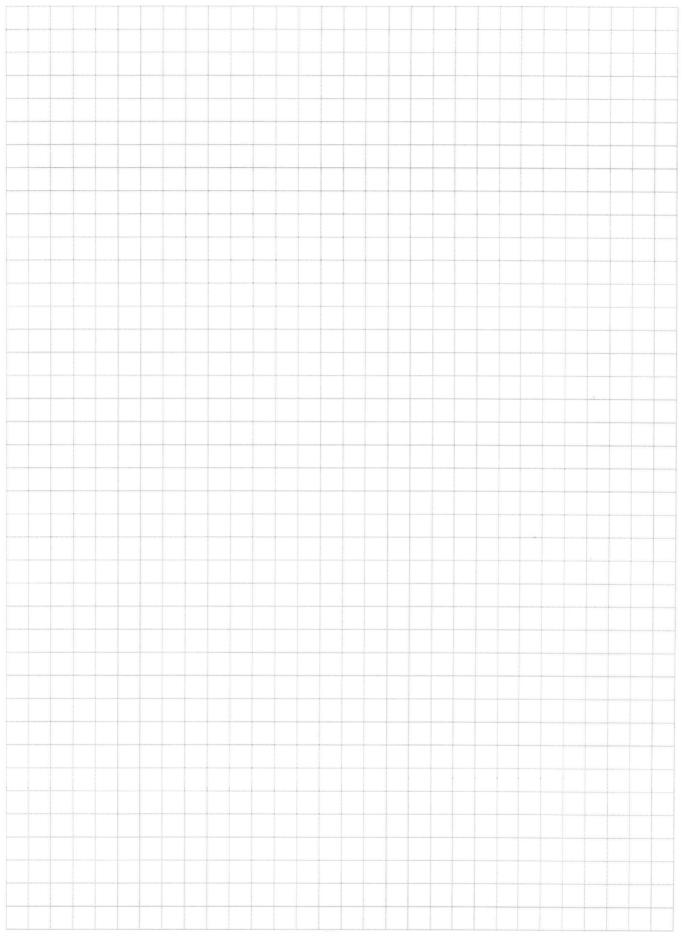

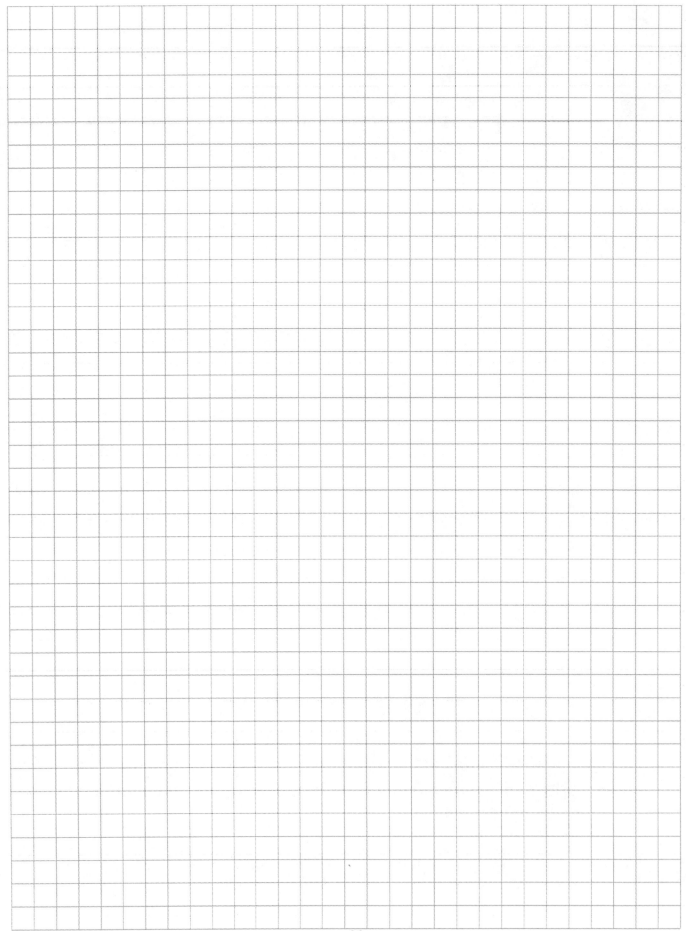

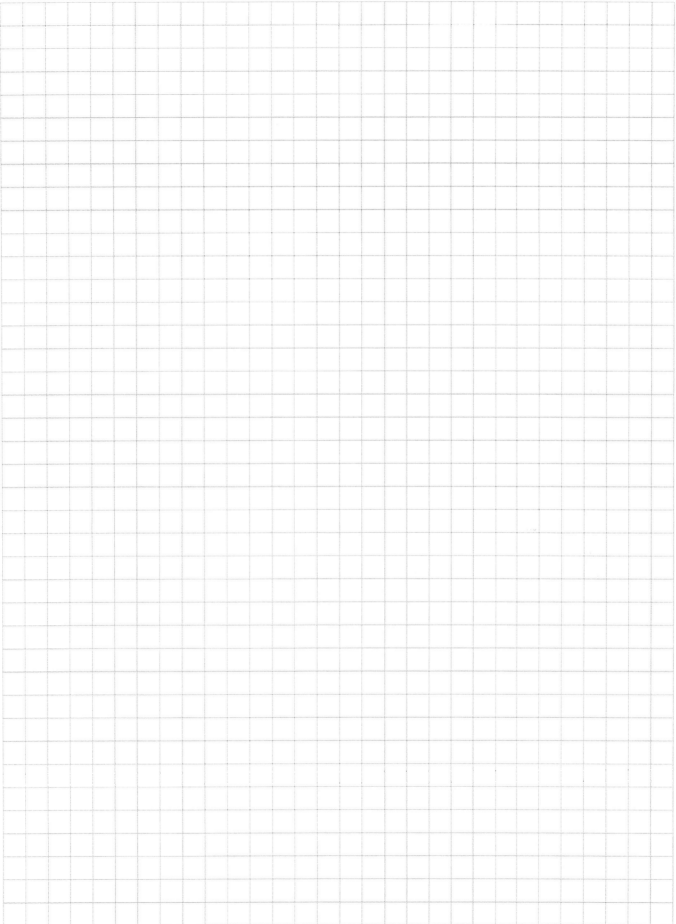

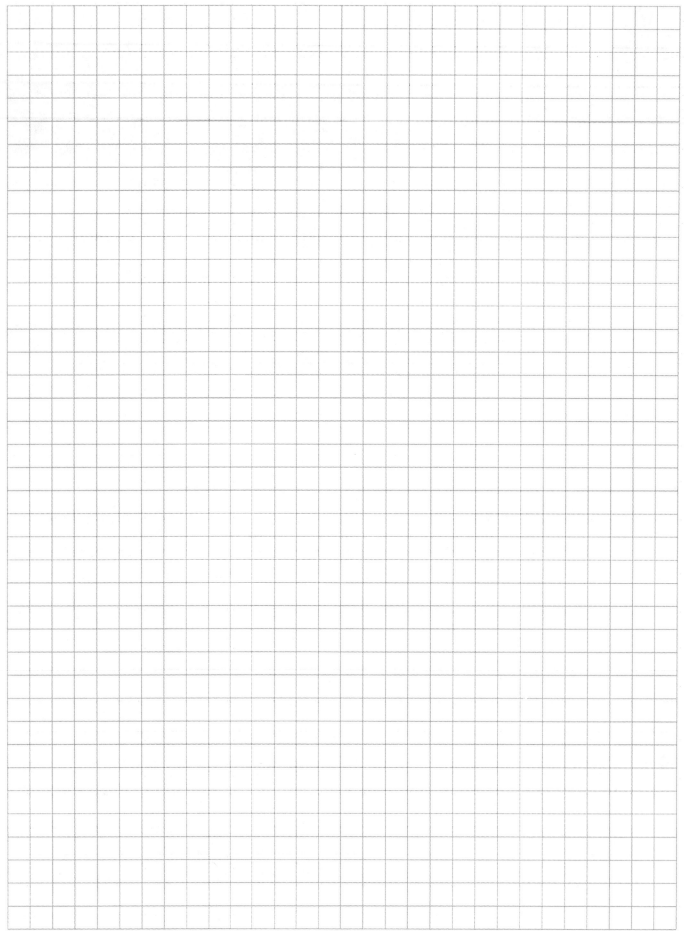

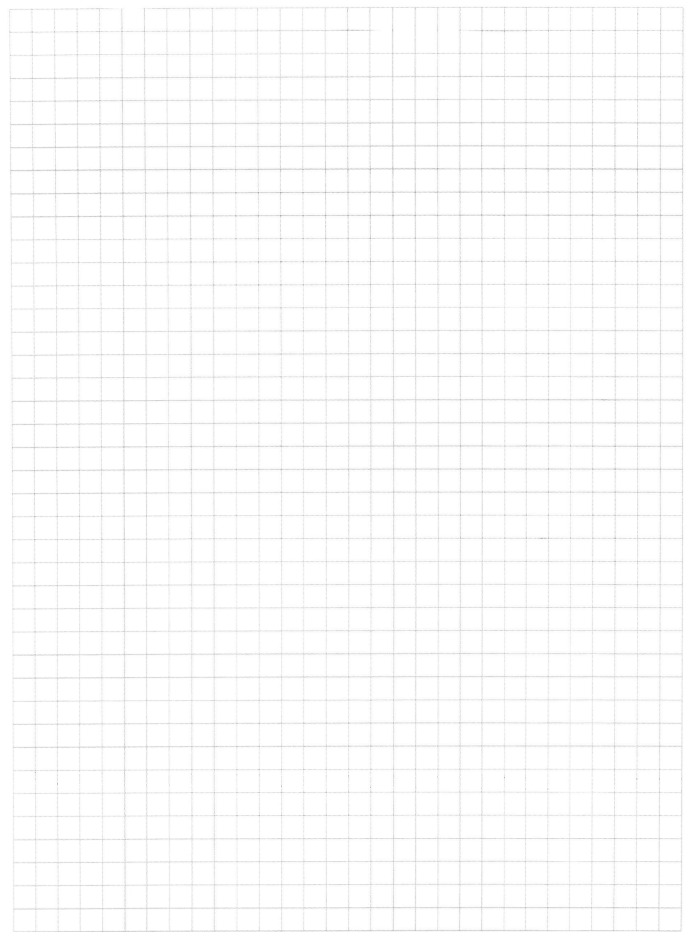

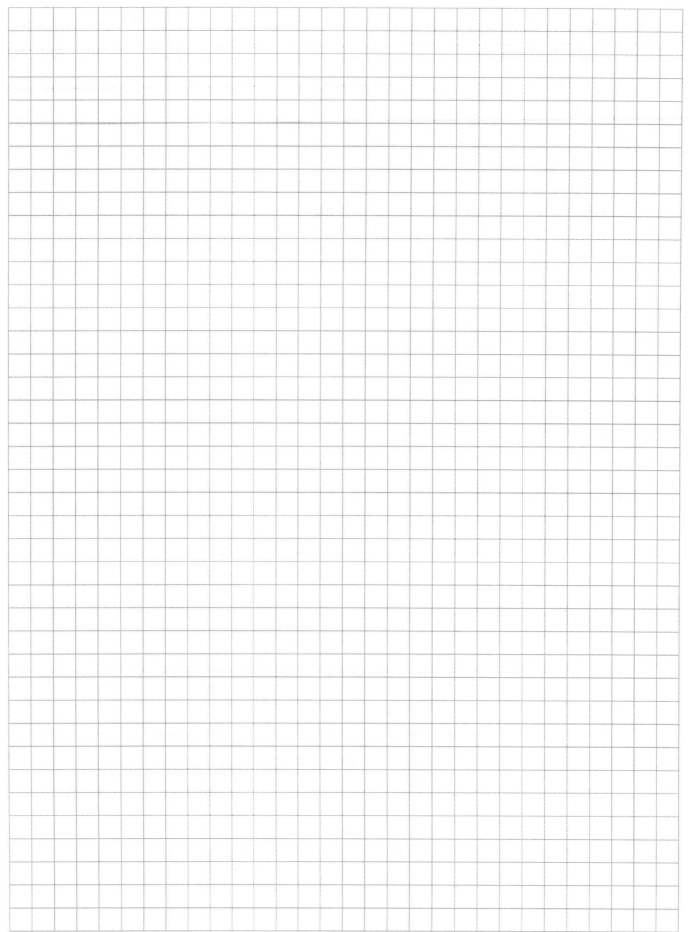

How did we do?

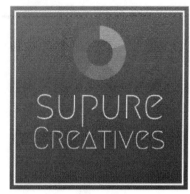

Good! Yeah... Please take some time to review us. It really helps our business and also other customers in making a decision. Thanks!

Not good! We're so sorry. Contact us: SupureCreatives@gmail.com & give us a chance to fix it...

Thank you for your support!
A portion of the proceeds will go to selected charity purpose (check our Author Page for details).

To submit a review:
1. Go to the product detail page for the item on Amazon.com. If you've placed an order for the item, you can also go to **Your Orders**
2. Click **Write a customer review** in the **Customer Reviews** section.
3. Select a **Star Rating**. A green check mark shows for successfully submitted ratings.
4. Add text, photos, or videos and click **Submit**. Thank you very much!

amazon.com/author/SupureCreatives

If you have any question - contact us: **SupureCreatives@gmail.com**

Made in the USA
Las Vegas, NV
07 October 2024

96434196R00057